Patient
Self-Management
of
Chronic Disease

Other Titles of Interest

Barbara K. Redman, PhD, RN, FAAN

Patient
Self-Management of
Chronic Disease

The Health Care Provider's Challenge

JONES AND BARTLETT PUBLISHERS

Sudbury, Massachusetts

BOSTON   TORONTO   LONDON   SINGAPORE

World Headquarters

Jones and Bartlett
Publishers
40 Tall Pine Drive
Sudbury, MA 01776
978-443-5000
info@jbpub.com
www.jbpub.com

Jones and Bartlett
Publishers Canada
2406 Nikanna Road
Mississauga, ON L5C
2W6
CANADA

Jones and Bartlett
Publishers International
Barb House, Barb Mews
London W6 7PA
UK

Production Credits
Acquisitions Editor: Penny M. Glynn
Associate Editor: Karen Zuck
Senior Production Editor: Julie C. Bolduc
Manufacturing Buyer: Amy Bacus
Associate Marketing Manager: Joy Stark-Vancs
Composition: Interactive Composition Corporation
Text Design: dcdesign
Cover Design: Kristin E. Ohlin
Cover Image: © Creatas
Printing and Binding: Malloy Lithographing
Cover Printing: Malloy Lithographing

Library of Congress Cataloging-in-Publication Data
Redman, Barbara Klug.
    Patient self-management of chronic disease : the health care
provider's challenge / Barbara K. Redman. -- 1st ed.
        p. ; cm.
Includes bibliographical references and index.
    ISBN 0-7637-2307-X (alk. paper)
1. Patient education.   2. Self care, Health.   3. Chronic
diseases--Treatment.
    [DNLM: 1. Chronic Disease.   2. Self Care.   3. Patient
Participation. WT 500 R318p 2004]   I. Title.
    R727.4.R427   2004
    615.5'071--dc21

Printed in the United States of America
07 06 05 04 03   10 9 8 7 6 5 4 3 2 1

Contents

Preface

Because of the unfortunate continued dominance of a narrow medical model, educational or skills training in chronic illness is still viewed as merely supportive as opposed to being a major therapeutic element in patient care. The premise of this book is that preparation for self-management (SM) is essential for patient and family safety, adaptation, and stress management and that such preparation must be constantly available throughout the course of the health problem, just as is drug therapy. In addition to ignoring SM, the medical model includes a strong emphasis on patient compliance with physician orders, an unfortunate and destructive value bias that ignores the patient's perspective.

The long-standing debate on compliance treats the provider's perspective as an uncontroversial point of departure, assuming first the propriety of treatment recommendations and second the irrelevance of patient and family goals. Health professionals' inability to value patient perspective and expertise frequently leads to a spiral of discrediting the patient's view, ridicule, dismissal, and mutual alienation. Under the medical model, health professionals have little appreciation for aspects of illness beyond what biomedical science makes rational. Failing to prioritize disease above all other life issues renders the patient vulnerable to accusations of noncompliance. So patients learn to pretend compliance (Thorne, Nyhlin, Paterson, 2000) and everyone else believes that the first goal is to get them to do what the physician says.

This interminable debate has diverted attention from the real issue: how, based on a negotiated set of treatment goals, to prepare patients and their caregivers for the monumental responsibilities they carry.

Today, considerable evidence suggests that most of the population is not receiving the SM preparation they need, even in areas where the evidence base for it is very strong. Availability of preparation for SM of various chronic diseases lies on a continuum from being well recognized and thoroughly studied to being virtually ignored. For example, even diabetes SM, the best-established, fails to reach large segments of the population in need; SM for epilepsy and multiple sclerosis, on the other hand, is virtually nonexistent even though strong evidence indicates that it is needed. For HIV/AIDS, nearly all education is preventive and virtually none is oriented to SM preparation, even though these needs are great. The psychological literature has largely focused on adaptation and coping, rather than on gaining the skills needed for SM. These patterns show that SM preparation is far from being recognized as the standard of care, a situation that could be described as ethically incomprehensible and even a case of abandonment by health professionals.

Nurses are the health professionals whose skills and philosophy of practice compel patient/family preparation for SM, and advance practice nurses commonly carry caseloads of individuals with chronic illness. Unfortunately, this philosophy of practice is constantly at odds with payment policy for health care. The purpose of this book is to draw attention to the absolute necessity of SM preparation for patients and families and to show how it can be accomplished.

Reference

Thorne, S. E., Nyhlin, K., Paterson, B. L. (2000). Attitudes toward patient expertise in chronic illness. *International Journal of Nursing Studies 37*, 303–311.

Patient
Self-Management
of
Chronic Disease

1

Self-Management Preparation in Chronic Illness

Background and Need

Chronic diseases — many disabling — introduce significant psychosocial challenges and adaptive demands for patients and families. In many cases, biomedical understanding is limited and no cure is available. Uncertainty about diagnosis, lack of clear treatment indications, dependence on professional expertise and biomedical technology, and the unavailability of specialized services must all be dealt with. Pain, fatigue, weakness, physical disability, cognitive deficits, and sexual dysfunction are common, and illness intrudes in many ways on life (Devins, Cameron, Edworthy, 2000).

Patient/family self-management (SM) of chronic disease has always been inevitable; what is new is that it may finally be recognized by a health care system whose delivery and financing mechanisms have for 80 years been geared toward management of acute illness (Fox, 1995). Planned preparation of patients for SM is widely recognized to have begun with diabetes, as this disease's treatment pattern requires daily — if not hourly — attention to diet, insulin, and exercise. The model for patient preparation for diabetes SM has progressed significantly since those early days, in part reflecting advances in medical management of the disease and in part acknowledging accumulation of an impressive body of research about outcomes of SM preparation and how it might best be designed.

Evidence-based SM preparation for other chronic diseases lagged considerably. In the 1980s the U.S. federal government invested in development of validated SM preparation for asthma, and a few years later an innovative model was developed for arthritis (Lorig, 1996). Yet for most chronic diseases, SM or preparation for it is not recognized. Instead, patients are seen as dull or recalcitrant if they do not comply precisely with the prescribed medical management, even though providers are often uncertain about treatment effectiveness or do not provide the recommended treatment.

These trends must be seen as a major health care system failing. Not only were these services not available, but the "compliance with prescribed regimen" mentality also alienated patients from their health care providers, devalued their own SM skills and the necessity to experiment to attain them, and created a blame-the-victim standoff between providers and patients. To deal effectively with chronic illness, patients must learn bodily cues, emotional triggers, and their own unique response patterns and must match their decisions with their own desired quality of life, rather than one predetermined by the health care system (Thorne, 1999).

In addition, the compliance approach assumes an ideal, normative self that sees a combination of self-discipline and productivity as behavior essential for good health. The willingness to work so as to enact an efficient bodily productivity and balance are seen as indices of proper control (Ferzacca, 2000). Many people do not live this way (for example, they do not engage in patterned ways of life such as three meals a day at fixed times), and SM according to this ideology will not be able to connect with these individuals.

The purpose of the compliance ideology seems to be to maintain physician control. Professionals frequently value disease information over quality of life and control access to information by discrediting, ridiculing, or dismissing patients' views and skills (Thorne, Nhylin, Paterson, 2000). Because of the adoption of this set of attitudes, patients and families have been harmed and the benefits of work and school productivity that can accompany adequate patient SM have been lost.

This book describes evidence-based best practices for patient/family SM preparation for a wide variety of diseases, illnesses, and symptoms for which it should be available. This initial chapter provides concise background information on essential elements of SM preparation and on measurement instruments to assess the need for SM and judge its outcome, details theories underlying SM, explains how to judge the strength of the research evidence validating it, and identifies the policy context that frames incentives, or lack of them, for providing this care.

Each chapter describes a disease or symptom or a cluster of diseases/symptoms for which SM is necessary, using the following format: standards for SM preparation, interventions that have been shown to be effective in yielding competent self-managers for populations with a variety of cultural backgrounds and literacy levels, and measurement instruments. Teaching materials are widely available through disease-oriented organizations, government agencies, commercial companies, and Internet sources and thus are not included here.

The broader purpose of this book is to stimulate further development of patient SM preparation as a mandatory component of chronic disease care. SM without adequate preparation is substandard care and unethical but apparently common. For example, surveys of managed care organizations have documented that substandard care of this sort is the norm for people with diabetes who do not use insulin (Daly, Leontos, 1999). Fifty to 80 percent of individuals with diabetes have significant knowledge and skill deficits, and ideal glycemic control is achieved in fewer than half of persons with type 2 diabetes (Norris, Engelgau, Narayan, 2001). Likewise, although well-documented SM programs exist for asthma, a survey of emergency rooms that treat many of these patients showed they do not offer SM preparation and that their patients frequently lack adequate primary care.

Concept and Structure of Self-Management Preparation

Living with a chronic disease creates three types of work for patients:

1. Work necessitated by the disease, such as taking medicine and maintaining therapeutic exercise regimens
2. Work of maintaining everyday life such as employment and family
3. Work of dealing with an altered view of the future, including changing life plans and the frustration, anger, and depression that results

Managing these symptoms, disability, emotional impact, complex medication regimens, and difficult lifestyle adjustments and obtaining helpful health care are necessary clusters of skills. SM preparation, therefore, requires assisting patient and family caregivers in gaining skills and developing the confidence to apply those skills on a day-to-day basis, including coping with changing roles and emotions (Lorig, 1996).

Patient SM involves use of both diagnostic and therapeutic techniques — self-assessment of symptoms and self-treatment consisting of lifestyle adaptations and medications. For example, diabetes SM has included both measurement of blood sugar levels and modification of insulin administration, eating, and exercise. Hypertension SM has involved primarily assessment (monitoring of blood pressure) without self-treatment. There should be evidence of two advantages from SM: (1) treatment should be more effective because adaptations do not have to wait for provider approval, and (2) empowerment of patients to incorporate their own preferences and control their lives should yield a better quality of life. The goal is to return the patient to maximal function.

SM preparation can be delivered in separate programs, frequently community-based, as in workplaces or pharmacies, payer groups or managed care organizations, or it can be based in hospitals, physician practices, or long-term care settings and/or integrated into clinical practice. Health professionals frequently need training to learn how to provide SM preparation. In the United Kingdom, this learning occurs at national training centers, and in other countries it leads to provider certification (Partridge, Hill, 2002).

While most programs are disease-specific, it is possible to incorporate patients with a variety of chronic diseases into a single SM preparation program, as the developmental tasks are much the same. A review of research about the experience of chronic illness found commonalities of profound fatigue, pain and suffering, and challenge to identity or self-concept. Stigmatizing illnesses such as epilepsy, or those with no accepted biological basis such as chronic fatigue syndrome, yield additional adjustment problems. Information about the experiences of individuals not of middle-class background or European descent and those with cognitive impairments, trouble communicating, or inability to read or write has not been available (Thorne, Paterson, 2000).

Lorig and others' (1999) chronic disease SM program (CDSMP) provides an example. Focus groups showed common issues across disease entities. Given that people aged 60 and older have an average of 2.2 chronic conditions, this approach of crossing disease entities is particularly relevant. The program was run with 831 participants and was community-based, peer-led, and based on self-efficacy (SE) theory.

Each session of the seven-week course is divided into several 15- to 20-minute segments that expanded on content from previous weeks. This structure gives participants a chance to go home, practice, and get feedback on their progress. To enhance effectiveness, each session ends with participants contracting to do one self-chosen activity during the coming week. Each session begins with a feedback session in which participants report on their progress or the problems they experienced in carrying out their SM goal during the week. When problems occur, other class members are asked for solutions; in this way, problem-solving skills are learned by the participants and practiced many times during the program. Fifteen to 20 percent of class time is spent on assisting patients to deal with negative emotions such as anger, fear, frustration, and depression. Through structured exercises, participants share these emotions and use problem-solving techniques to find solutions.

CDSMP content is typical: exercise; cognitive symptom management techniques such as guided relaxation and distraction; nutrition; fatigue and sleep management; use of medications; use of community resources; managing emotions of fear, anger, and depression; and health-related problem solving and decision making. Besides the weekly action planning and feedback, this program uses modeling of behaviors, problem solving, and reinterpretation of symptoms. CDSMP includes the right instructional elements to increase SE (skills mastery through contracting and feedback, modeling by peer leaders, and making small continual changes through verbal persuasion and reinforcement) and to build problem-solving skills (instruction in how to deal with problems and practice in doing so).

A randomized controlled trial (RCT) of CDSMP showed improvements for the intervention group relative to the control group at six months in several parameters: amount of exercise; frequency of cognitive symptom management; self-reported health distress, fatigue, disability, and social/role activities limitation; and fewer hospitalizations and days in the hospital (Lorig and others, 1999). A follow-up study (Lorig et al., 2001) found that, compared with baseline, emergency room/outpatient visits and health distress were reduced and SE improved with the CDSMP.

Many other examples of SM preparation programs will be cited in the chapters to follow. Caregivers are also essential to patients' ability to self-manage chronic illness. A meta-analysis of multiple studies of the effectiveness of various kinds of interventions with caregivers found that psychoeducation had a significant effect on the care recipients' symptoms; caregiver burden, depression, and well-being; and on patient ability/knowledge. Longer interventions were more beneficial in alleviating care recipients' symptoms (seven to nine sessions) and caregiver depression (more than nine sessions) (Sorensen, Pinquart, Habil, Duberstein, 2002).

Learning Approaches

Four major learning theories/models have been used in effective SM preparation.

First is social learning theory, and especially the part of the theory that deals with SE (confidence that one can carry out elements of SM). SE is highly predictive of motivation and actual performance of SM. Its development in a patient is accomplished by performance attainments, vicarious experiences that involve observing others like oneself be successful, verbal persuasion, and perceived physiological states from which individuals partly judge their capability, strength, and vulnerability. Instruments for measuring SE for many SM behaviors are available. For example, the Self-Management of Heart Failure instrument is used to assess these patients' ability to monitor their symptoms and judge which need to be addressed immediately. One group of heart failure patients was self-managing treatment but was not matched to the correct symptom and had a considerable lack of self-confidence in managing the precarious balance between relative health and symptomatic heart failure (Riegel, Carlson, Glaser, 2000).

A second relevant theory is the transtheoretical model. It holds that intentional change requires movement through discrete motivational stages: precontemplation for considering changes, contemplation, preparation for change, taking action to change, and maintenance of change (Prochaska, Velicer, 1997).

Third, belief models have proved useful. The construct of patient-perceived barriers to SM, derived from the Health Belief Model, has been found to be strongly associated with following SM practices. Understanding patients' cognitive models of their illness — what caused it, what its consequences are, what its course will be, how effective treatment is — is necessary because this model guides their actions, including coping, adherence, and self-evaluation. The Implicit Models of Illness Questionnaire (IMIQ) is used to assess patient illness representations (Figure 1.1). IMIQ has a four-factor structure: curability, responsibility, symptom variability, and consequence. It was tested with persons with rheumatoid arthritis. Those who saw their arthritis as curable or who saw themselves as responsible for the illness reported a significant increase in depression over time, supporting construct validity of the instrument (Schiaffino, Cea, 1995). IMIQ has also been used with symptoms other than pain.

Implicit Models of Illness Questionnaire

Name:_ Date:_ _ _ _ _ _ _ _ _ _ _ _ _ _ _

It is important for us to learn more about your understanding of your pain problem (disease, diagnosis, pain symptoms). Please respond to each of the following statements about your pain problem(s). Please record your answers by placing an "x" on each of the scales below to indicate your level of agreement or disagreement with each statement about your pain problem.

1. My pain is controllable.

   Strongly _ _ _ _:_ _ _ _:_ _ _ _:_ _ _ _:_ _ _ _:_ _ _ _:_ _ _ _:_ _ _ _ Strongly
   Agree   Disagree

2. My pain requires medical attention.

   Strongly _ _ _ _:_ _ _ _:_ _ _ _:_ _ _ _:_ _ _ _:_ _ _ _:_ _ _ _:_ _ _ _ Strongly
   Agree   Disagree

3. My pain is chronic (long-lasting) rather than acute (short-lived).

   Strongly _ _ _ _:_ _ _ _:_ _ _ _:_ _ _ _:_ _ _ _:_ _ _ _:_ _ _ _:_ _ _ _ Strongly
   Agree   Disagree

4. A symptom of my pain is fever.

   Strongly _ _ _ _:_ _ _ _:_ _ _ _:_ _ _ _:_ _ _ _:_ _ _ _:_ _ _ _:_ _ _ _ Strongly
   Agree   Disagree

5. My pain is disabling.

   Strongly _ _ _ _:_ _ _ _:_ _ _ _:_ _ _ _:_ _ _ _:_ _ _ _:_ _ _ _:_ _ _ _ Strongly
   Agree   Disagree

6. My pain seems to be located in the area of my stomach (abdomen, intestinal tract).

   Strongly _ _ _ _:_ _ _ _:_ _ _ _:_ _ _ _:_ _ _ _:_ _ _ _:_ _ _ _:_ _ _ _ Strongly
   Agree   Disagree

7. My pain is cured or greatly relieved by pain-killers (drugs, medicine).

   Strongly _ _ _ _:_ _ _ _:_ _ _ _:_ _ _ _:_ _ _ _:_ _ _ _:_ _ _ _:_ _ _ _ Strongly
   Agree   Disagree

8. My pain has serious consequences for me.

   Strongly _ _ _ _:_ _ _ _:_ _ _ _:_ _ _ _:_ _ _ _:_ _ _ _:_ _ _ _:_ _ _ _ Strongly
   Agree   Disagree

FIGURE 1.1

9. My pain is caused (made worse) by changes in the weather.

Strongly _ _ _ _:_ _ _ _:_ _ _ _:_ _ _ _:_ _ _ _:_ _ _ _:_ _ _ _:_ _ _ _:_ _ _ _ Strongly
Agree   Disagree

10. My pain seems to be on the surface of my skin.

Strongly _ _ _ _:_ _ _ _:_ _ _ _:_ _ _ _:_ _ _ _:_ _ _ _:_ _ _ _:_ _ _ _:_ _ _ _ Strongly
Agree   Disagree

11. My pain is excruciating.

Strongly _ _ _ _:_ _ _ _:_ _ _ _:_ _ _ _:_ _ _ _:_ _ _ _:_ _ _ _:_ _ _ _:_ _ _ _ Strongly
Agree   Disagree

12. My pain symptoms are similar to the symptoms of a cold.

Strongly _ _ _ _:_ _ _ _:_ _ _ _:_ _ _ _:_ _ _ _:_ _ _ _:_ _ _ _:_ _ _ _:_ _ _ _ Strongly
Agree   Disagree

13. My pain requires hospitalization.

Strongly _ _ _ _:_ _ _ _:_ _ _ _:_ _ _ _:_ _ _ _:_ _ _ _:_ _ _ _:_ _ _ _:_ _ _ _ Strongly
Agree   Disagree

14. My pain is permanent rather than temporary.

Strongly _ _ _ _:_ _ _ _:_ _ _ _:_ _ _ _:_ _ _ _:_ _ _ _:_ _ _ _:_ _ _ _:_ _ _ _ Strongly
Agree   Disagree

15. My pain is less intense when stress is reduced.

Strongly _ _ _ _:_ _ _ _:_ _ _ _:_ _ _ _:_ _ _ _:_ _ _ _:_ _ _ _:_ _ _ _:_ _ _ _ Strongly
Agree   Disagree

16. My pain is caused (made much worse) by stress or nerves.

Strongly _ _ _ _:_ _ _ _:_ _ _ _:_ _ _ _:_ _ _ _:_ _ _ _:_ _ _ _:_ _ _ _:_ _ _ _ Strongly
Agree   Disagree

17. Sometimes my pain goes away on its own.

Strongly _ _ _ _:_ _ _ _:_ _ _ _:_ _ _ _:_ _ _ _:_ _ _ _:_ _ _ _:_ _ _ _:_ _ _ _ Strongly
Agree   Disagree

18. My pain is caused by my own behavior (things that I do).

Strongly _ _ _ _:_ _ _ _:_ _ _ _:_ _ _ _:_ _ _ _:_ _ _ _:_ _ _ _:_ _ _ _:_ _ _ _ Strongly
Agree   Disagree

FIGURE 1.1 *(continued)*

19. My pain is constant.

Strongly _ _ _:_ _ _:_ _ _:_ _ _:_ _ _:_ _ _:_ _ _:_ _ _:_ _ _ Strongly
Agree   Disagree

20. My pain is greatly reduced by eating properly.

Strongly _ _ _:_ _ _:_ _ _:_ _ _:_ _ _:_ _ _:_ _ _:_ _ _:_ _ _ Strongly
Agree   Disagree

21. I can do some things to control my pain.

Strongly _ _ _:_ _ _:_ _ _:_ _ _:_ _ _:_ _ _:_ _ _:_ _ _:_ _ _ Strongly
Agree   Disagree

22. My pain is greatly reduced by rest.

Strongly _ _ _:_ _ _:_ _ _:_ _ _:_ _ _:_ _ _:_ _ _:_ _ _:_ _ _ Strongly
Agree   Disagree

23. My pain problems developed because of something I did.

Strongly _ _ _:_ _ _:_ _ _:_ _ _:_ _ _:_ _ _:_ _ _:_ _ _:_ _ _ Strongly
Agree   Disagree

24. My symptoms are contagious.

Strongly _ _ _:_ _ _:_ _ _:_ _ _:_ _ _:_ _ _:_ _ _:_ _ _:_ _ _ Strongly
Agree   Disagree

25. My pain changes with the seasons of the year.

Strongly _ _ _:_ _ _:_ _ _:_ _ _:_ _ _:_ _ _:_ _ _:_ _ _:_ _ _ Strongly
Agree   Disagree

26. My pain is caused by germs or virus.

Strongly _ _ _:_ _ _:_ _ _:_ _ _:_ _ _:_ _ _:_ _ _:_ _ _:_ _ _ Strongly
Agree   Disagree

27. My pain is made much worse by lack of rest.

Strongly _ _ _:_ _ _:_ _ _:_ _ _:_ _ _:_ _ _:_ _ _:_ _ _:_ _ _ Strongly
Agree   Disagree

28. My pain can be avoided or greatly reduced.

Strongly _ _ _:_ _ _:_ _ _:_ _ _:_ _ _:_ _ _:_ _ _:_ _ _:_ _ _ Strongly
Agree   Disagree

FIGURE 1.1 (continued)

29. My pain is serious.

Strongly _ _ _:_ _ _:_ _ _:_ _ _:_ _ _:_ _ _:_ _ _:_ _ _:_ _ _:_ _ _ Strongly
Agree   Disagree

30. Even if it goes away for a while, my pain always comes back.

Strongly _ _ _:_ _ _:_ _ _:_ _ _:_ _ _:_ _ _:_ _ _:_ _ _:_ _ _:_ _ _ Strongly
Agree   Disagree

31. No one is responsible for the onset of my pain.

Strongly _ _ _:_ _ _:_ _ _:_ _ _:_ _ _:_ _ _:_ _ _:_ _ _:_ _ _:_ _ _ Strongly
Agree   Disagree

32. The intensity (severity) of my pain varies.

Strongly _ _ _:_ _ _:_ _ _:_ _ _:_ _ _:_ _ _:_ _ _:_ _ _:_ _ _:_ _ _ Strongly
Agree   Disagree

33. My pain is caused or made worse by poor diet.

Strongly _ _ _:_ _ _:_ _ _:_ _ _:_ _ _:_ _ _:_ _ _:_ _ _:_ _ _:_ _ _ Strongly
Agree   Disagree

34. My pain is curable.

Strongly _ _ _:_ _ _:_ _ _:_ _ _:_ _ _:_ _ _:_ _ _:_ _ _:_ _ _:_ _ _ Strongly
Agree   Disagree

35. My pain varies (changes) over time.

Strongly _ _ _:_ _ _:_ _ _:_ _ _:_ _ _:_ _ _:_ _ _:_ _ _:_ _ _:_ _ _ Strongly
Agree   Disagree

36. My pain seems to be located in my head.

Strongly _ _ _:_ _ _:_ _ _:_ _ _:_ _ _:_ _ _:_ _ _:_ _ _:_ _ _:_ _ _ Strongly
Agree   Disagree

37. My pain affects many parts of my body.

Strongly _ _ _:_ _ _:_ _ _:_ _ _:_ _ _:_ _ _:_ _ _:_ _ _:_ _ _:_ _ _ Strongly
Agree   Disagree

38. My pain is greatly reduced by physical exercise.

Strongly _ _ _:_ _ _:_ _ _:_ _ _:_ _ _:_ _ _:_ _ _:_ _ _:_ _ _:_ _ _ Strongly
Agree   Disagree

FIGURE 1.1 (continued)

Petrie, Cameron, Ellis, Buick, and Weinman (2002) found that patients who believed their myocardial infarction would have more serious long-lasting consequences had greater levels of illness-related disability and were slower to return to work than those who did not have such beliefs. Patients with such beliefs can be identified early after myocardial infarction onset. Petrie et al.'s study used the patient's own model of his or her illness initially but then challenged false and highly negative ideas, such as the belief that the patient would need to significantly reduce activities over the long term. A written recovery plan was developed and personalized to each patient's particular circumstances for return to work, with an explicit plan of exercise and dietary change. The intervention significantly altered patients' beliefs about the illness, converting their perspective to one that their heart condition could be controlled. Formal cardiac rehabilitation programs may or may not incorporate this and other important theoretical perspectives.

The fourth important learning perspective/theory is that of problem solving. It and its associated interventions are explained in the next section on SM preparation approaches.

Some might consider the theory of planned behavior to be a fifth useful theory for SM preparation. It has been touted as beneficial in establishing a strong intention to change behavior among people who may lack it. This theory is an extension of the theory of reasoned action, which states that the proximal determinant of behavior is an intention to act. This intention is influenced by the individual's attitude toward a behavior, subjective norm, and perceived behavioral control. Hardeman and others' (2002) overview of the evidence found few coherent studies that were explicit about how this theory had been applied and little use of this theory to develop or evaluate interventions, leaving insufficient evidence to judge its relevance to SM.

In practice, these learning theories are used together. The nature of the SM issue to be solved will guide selection of the most relevant theories, sometimes in a particular learning framework. For example, *constructivists* posit that knowledge is constructed, not transmitted, and that the construction occurs from activity in a context. Table 1.1 contrasts constructivist

TABLE 1.1 Constructivist Versus Traditional Learning Methods

	Constructivist	**Traditional**
Knowledge	Constructed, emergent, situated in action or experience, distributed	Transmitted, external to knower, objective, stable, fixed, decontextualized
Reality	Product of mind	External to the knower
Meaning	Reflects perceptions and understanding of experiences	Reflects external world
Symbols	Tools for constructing reality	Represents world
Learning	Knowledge construction, interpreting world, constructing meaning, ill-structured, authentic-experiential, articulation-reflection, process-oriented	Knowledge transmission, reflecting what teacher knows, well-structured, abstract-symbolic, encoding-retention-retrieval, product-oriented
Instruction	Reflecting multiple perspectives, increasing complexity, diversity, bottom-up, inductive, apprenticeship, modeling, coaching, exploration, learner-generated	Simplify knowledge, abstract rules, basics first, top-down, deductive, application of symbols (rules, principles), lecturing, tutoring, instructor derived and controlled, individual, competitive

Source: Jonassen, D. H., Peck, K. L., Wilson, B. G. (1999). *Learning with Technology.* Columbus, OH: Merrill. Reprinted by permission of Pearson Education, Inc., Upper Saddle River, NJ.

and traditional learning methods. Under traditional methods, novices are trained to work on problems that are decontextualized and well structured; in everyday life, however, problems are complex and ill structured, with no clear beginning and end, many possible solution paths, and many subproblems

(Jonassen, Peck, Wilson, 1999). Constructivists would argue that traditional learning methods are not an effective or efficient way to create self-managers, who must solve real problems every day.

Constructivists would advocate teaching methods not typically used by traditionalists. For example, when we learn how to use a skill, we remember it as a story. We later recall those stories when faced with similar experiences and attempt to use them to guide activities. Stories elicited from skilled problem solvers indexed for the lessons they have to teach and made available to learners in case libraries can support problem-solving instruction with a constructivist bent (Jonassen, Hernandez-Serrano, 2002).

Other learning conditions are important as well for many patients with chronic illness, who may also have a cognitive deficiency. Frequently these patients are overwhelmed by the amount to learn and are helped by decreasing the cognitive load (Van Gerven, Paas, Van Meerienboer, Schmidt, 2000). Time pressure, task complexity, and environmental noise can all increase cognitive load and overwhelm working memory capacity. This load can be reduced by focusing only on absolutely germane issues and by breaking complex tasks into several simple subtasks. An additional way to decrease load is to build a patient's schemas, incorporating lower-level schemas into a more comprehensive one, which is easily transferred to other learning situations and therefore well remembered. A schema can be anything that has been learned and treated as a single entity; if learning has occurred over a long period of time, a schema may incorporate a huge amount of information (Kirschner, 2002).

Self-Management Preparation Approaches

The wide range of teaching approaches reviewed in basic texts for patient education (Redman, 2001) is also appropriate for SM preparation but must be clearly focused on SM and not on simpler goals of information learning. Because no agreed-upon taxonomy for classifying intervention types exists, verbal descriptions of the teaching approach, learner activities, goals and outcomes, and length of contact time are used to describe (somewhat imprecisely) the intervention.

In addition to assessments of well-established teaching and coaching approaches, evidence is still accumulating for new approaches. For example, decision aids are designed to assist consumers in making a particular health decision (such as whether to use hormone replacement therapy or which treatment approach to use for prostate cancer), providing information in functional terms and in probabilities related to alternatives, benefits, and risks. Each decision aid uses information tailored to a patient's clinical risk profile and explicitly asks patients to consider what they value most highly. A review of RCTs testing decision aids found some improved outcomes but insufficient evidence to judge the considerable cost of their development (Estabrooks and others, 2001).

Internet-based SM programs, which are particularly useful for patients in rural areas and homebound patients, are just beginning to be tested. One such program for diabetes tracked blood glucose levels and provided direction for physical activity and communication with other participants (McKay, King, Eaking, Seeley, Glasgow, 2001).

SM education must address a set of learning tasks different from those in other areas of patient education, such as acute symptom management. For example, many patients do not initially understand that no cure for their disease exists and assume that medical and self-management will yield a complete remission. They also do not understand that providers are often uncertain about the course of their chronic illness and the ability of a given treatment to control it. Providers can merely guess at what will be the best fit for a given patient with the disorder, making a trial-and-error process of adjusting treatment often necessary. This variability means that patients must learn to accept uncertainty both intellectually and emotionally. The probabilistic nature of the disease and its management is emphasized throughout SM education (Caplin, Creer, 2001).

Long-term maintenance of SM skills over time and across settings is, of course, a desired outcome of preparation but has been little studied to date. Caplin and Creer's work with adults with asthma shows that those who abandoned SM practice lacked commitment to strengthen their SE so that they could make life changes and gain control over their asthma. Those who had honed the sophisticated intellectual sequence of monitoring their disease, processing and evaluating data, making decisions, and taking action sustained their SM, as did those with a wide range of behavioral skills for coping with their disease. Because most patients acquire their SM skills when they are asymptomatic, they need repreated assessment and refinement of those skills when they must actually be used (Caplin, Creer, 2001).

Definition of appropriate outcomes, levels of achievement considered adequate, and measures have proved problematic. Diabetes SM is an example (Peeples, Mulcahy, Tomley, Weaver, 2001). It has focused primarily on evaluating the structure and process of education, with outcomes remaining poorly defined. Glycolated hemoglobin, body mass index, and lipid levels have been used as outcome measurements but are also strongly impacted by medical management, which may be substandard. Outcomes more specific to SM preparation must be identified.

Problem-Solving Framework/Skills

In chronic illness, psychological and physical health is largely dependent on the individual's ability to thoughtfully plan routines of diet, activity, and medication, regardless of competing life demands, stressors, or temporal moods. These SM tasks require problem-solving skills frequently not incorporated in traditional patient education. A problem exists when no effective response is apparent or available. Problems are novel, ambiguous, uncertain, with conflicting demands and lack of resources. An effective solution achieves the goal while minimizing negative consequences. Problem-centered instruction can be contrasted with the more usual topic-centered instruction.

The familiar process of defining problems, generating alternatives, deciding on a solution, and implementing and monitoring effectiveness must be taught and practiced to the level of competence in all areas of SM. Patients must understand these steps, have solving of relevant problems modeled for them, and practice solving problems with feedback on how well they did. At stage 1, learners solve problems by analogy, referring to known examples and relating them to the problems to be solved. At stage 2, they develop rules that guide their problem solving. At stage 3, problem-solving performance becomes smooth and rapid. At stage 4, learners who have practiced resolution of many different types of problems can retrieve a solution quickly from memory. Demonstating problem solving is instructionally more effective than telling how it might be done. It is also important to learn how to recognize an error, how to recover from it, and how to avoid the error in the future. Coaching in how to solve the problem is gradually withdrawn.

The general learning literature contains a body of research on using worked examples as instructional devices for learners to study. This approach provides an expert's problem solution with multiple examples of the kinds of problems that learners are likely to encounter; the examples are especially helpful in early stages of skill development in problem solving. Worked examples typically include a problem statement and a procedure for solving the problem and can decrease trial-and-error learning by providing a model of how to solve a set of problems (Atkinson, Derry, Renkl, Wortham, 2000).

Memory organization (also called knowledge structure, mental models, or schemas) is important for the kind of retrieval needed for problem solving. Knowledge structures that develop toward those of experts yield enhanced capability to make inferences, predict future events, and determine optimal actions more quickly and yield more complete comprehension.

Equally important is warding off negative emotions such as frustration, anxiety, and depression. Patients with these emotions who are unskilled at problem solving avoid problems or solve them impulsively with a lack of confidence. Elevated negative orientation may override the beneficial attributes of good problem-solving abilities (Elliott, Shewchuk, Miller, Richards, 2001). Also, all of this training must usually be spread over a prolonged period of time and continued with active practice to the point of mastery, so these skills will automatically "kick in" when the individual is under stress. For example, cancer patients who were less effective problem solvers reported higher levels of anxiety and depression as well as more cancer-related problems (Nezu et al., 1999).

As indicated earlier, caregiver families need all of the above-mentioned supports as well. Problem-solving abilities are associated with caregiver adjustment and are predictive of care recipients' psychosocial adjustment and medical complications (Elliott, Shewchuk, 2000). A RCT of a problem-solving skills training intervention for the mothers of newly diagnosed pediatric cancer patients provides an especially important example, as the emotional adjustment of such children is directly related to that of their parents (Sahler and others, 2002). This intervention included a current problem-solving inventory, worksheets at each session to structure the problem-solving process, and homework to identify and solve a problem. Direct instruction plus coaching, modeling, rehearsal, performance feedback, reinforcement, and shaping were used.

In summary, strong evidence suggests (1) that SM programs must contain solid skills in problem solving and development of clinical judgment, SE building, skills development, and belief modification and symptom reinterpretation as necessary, and (2) that stage-based theories such as the transtheoretical model are often helpful in this regard. Periodic assessment of the levels of these skills and sustained attention to patient competencies are necessary. Populations most affected by chronic conditions — the elderly, minorities, the poor, and patients with low levels of formal education — are dually affected by the potentially decreased cognitive functioning that accompanies their disease and by problems with health literacy. While many tests of SE and of knowledge are available, standard ways to assess problem-solving skills and judgment for SM remain rare.

A summary of research on the needs of parents of children with chronic illness shows need for (1) normality and certainty, which can be accomplished through management of illness; (2) information; and (3) partnership and recognition of their expertise in management of their child, in part to retain control and minimize uncertainty. Many parents are dissatisfied with the information they can get and believe they are not treated as partners (Fisher, 2001).

Rating the Evidence and Estimating the Need

The practice guidelines movement has emphasized the need to shift from a historical reliance on professional opinion to collection of rigorous scientific evidence of treatment effectiveness. This movement has also standardized ratings of quality of research evidence about a particular clinical issue and its summary into a usable judgment about which professional interventions should be supported and which should be abandoned because they do not yield useful outcomes. The issue of how to judge what counts as evidence and what weight to assign to different kinds of evidence is addressed by Hadorn and colleagues (1996).

An observed effect (or lack of effect) in studies may be biased by data collection methods and/or analysis and by failure to account for confounding variables. Research methodologists agree that the threat of bias is strongest in case reports and expert opinion, next strongest in case series and registries, case control studies, and cohort studies, and least vulnerable to bias in RCTs. Small sample size and conduct of a study in a single institution also increase probability of bias. Table 1.2 describes the quality of evidence from strongest to weakest. Many experts cluster 1–3 into level A, group 4–6 into level B, and reserve level C for expert opinion.

Meta-analyses (MA) provide statistical integration of findings from multiple studies. MA can vary in quality, however, with the strongest systematically including all relevant articles, incorporating some measure of study quality, and being done according to standards. A MA of RCTs can be ranked as evidence level 1 or 2 in Table 1.2, depending on sample size. A well-conducted MA of cohort studies was ranked at level 3. A MA showing a trend that did not reach statistical significance should be considered equivalent to several studies giving conflicting results (level 6 evidence).

Table 1.3 details well-recognized elements in study design and execution that affect validity and both major and minor flaws. A major flaw creates a potential for bias large enough to overturn a study's results; Hadorn and others (1996) considered three minor flaws to be equivalent to a major flaw. In each

TABLE 1.2   Level of Evidence for Guideline Recommendations

1. Supportive evidence from well-conducted randomized controlled trials that included 100 patients or more

   a. Evidence from a well-conducted multicenter trial

   b. Evidence from a meta-analysis that incorporated quality ratings in the analysis and included a total of 100 patients in its estimate of effect size and confidence intervals

2. Supportive evidence from well-conducted randomized controlled trials that included fewer than 100 patients

   a. Evidence from a well-conducted trial at one or more institutions

   b. Evidence from a meta-analysis that incorporated quality ratings in the analysis and included fewer than 100 patients in its estimate of effect size and confidence intervals

3. Supportive evidence from well-conducted cohort studies

   a. Evidence from a well-conducted prospective cohort study or registry

   b. Evidence from a well-conducted retrospective cohort study

   c. Evidence from a well-conducted meta-analysis of cohort studies

4. Supportive evidence from a well-conducted case-control study

5. Supportive evidence from poorly controlled or uncontrolled studies

   a. Evidence from randomized clinical trials with one or more major or three or more minor methodological flaws that could invalidate the results

   b. Evidence from observational studies with high potential for bias (such as case series with comparison to historical controls)

   c. Evidence from case series or case reports

6. Conflicting evidence with the weight of evidence supporting the recommendation

7. Expert opinion

Source: Hadorn, D. C., Baker, D., Hodges, J. S., Hicks, N. (1996). Rating the quality of evidence for clinical practice guidelines. *Journal of Clinical Epidemiology 49,* 749–754.

TABLE 1.3   Quality Assessment Criteria

1. Selection of Patients

Major Flaws

a. The diagnostic criteria for the disease under study were not described.

b. The criteria for admission to and exclusion from the study were not specified.

c. The decision regarding inclusion or exclusion from the study was sometimes made after treatment was initiated.

d. The study population was not representative of the majority of patients with the condition under investigation.

e. For cohort studies, the study groups were not treated concurrently.

Minor Flaws

a. The diagnostic criteria for the disease under study were inadequately described.

b. The criteria for admission to and exclusion from the study were inadequately described.

c. Patients were excluded from participation in the study, but no list or table of the reasons for exclusion was given.

2. Allocation of Patients to Treatment Groups

RANDOMIZED CLINICAL TRIALS

Major Flaws

a. Statements in the paper suggest that patients were not randomly assigned.

b. Known prognostic factors or confounders for the outcome of interest were not measured at baseline, or there was no comparison of the values for these variables for the study groups.

Minor Flaw

Patients were not allocated to the study groups in a truly randomized fashion (e.g., randomization by birth date, every other patient given placebo).

(continued)

TABLE 1.3 (continued)

COHORT OR REGISTRY STUDIES

Major Flaw

Known prognostic factors for the outcome of interest or possible confounders were not measured at baseline.

Minor Flaws

None

3. Therapeutic Regimen

Major Flaws

None

Minor Flaws

a. The mean daily dose actually taken by patients during the trial was not recorded.

b. The actual dosing schedule was not described and only the total daily dose is given.

c. Titration end points were not described.

d. Other therapeutic maneuvers were not described adequately enough that the study could be repeated.

4. Study Administration

Major Flaws

a. Patients were crossed over into the other group outside of the study design.

b. Medications were used that were not part of the original study design.

c. Other breaks in the study protocol occurred.

Minor Flaw

In a multicenter study, methods of diagnosis, treatment, or outcome measurement were not identical among the participating centers.

(continued)

TABLE 1.3 (continued)

5. Withdrawals from the Study

Major Flaws

a. Patients withdrew from the study, and the reasons for withdrawal were not listed. This includes an unexplained reduction in the number of patients recorded in the tables.

b. Sensitivity analysis shows that the number of withdrawals with unknown or unlisted outcomes could significantly bias the results. For example, if three patients in the treatment group who were lost to follow-up or not recorded had actually died, a significant reduction in mortality in the treated group would be made insignificant.

Minor Flaw

There was an excessive number of withdrawals regardless of the reasons: 10% for studies lasting less than three months or more than 15% for studies lasting for more than three months.

6. Patient Blinding (Randomized Controlled Trials Only)

Major Flaws

a. A placebo was not used for the control group.

b. For a study that used patient self-reported health status or symptoms as an end point, a study that claimed to be placebo controlled gave no description of how the placebo was administered.

Minor Flaws

a. For a study that used mortality as an end point, a study that claimed to be placebo controlled gave no description of how the placebo was administered.

b. For a study that used patient self-reported health status or symptoms as an end point, the physical characteristics, side effects, or method of administration of the placebo differed from that of the active drug so that it was possible for the patient to discern the treatment assignment.

(continued)

TABLE 1.3 (continued)

7. Outcome Measurement

Major Flaws

a. For a study that required investigators to rate patient clinical status or measure clinical parameters, the investigators were not blinded to the patient treatment group. (Double-blind methodology was not used.)

b. For a study that required investigators to rate patient clinical status or measure clinical parameters, the method of administration or the effects of the study drug and the placebo differed enough that investigators were likely to guess the patient treatment. (Double-blind methodology was attempted, but it suffered from serious flaws.)

Minor Flaws

a. For a study that measured mortality, the investigators were not blinded to the patient treatment group. (Double-blind methodology was not used.)

b. For a study that measured mortality, the method of administration or the effects of the study drug and the placebo differed enough that investigators were likely to guess the patient treatment. (Double-blind methodology was attempted, but it suffered from serious flaws.)

8. Statistical Analysis

Major Flaws

a. The analytical techniques described are incorrect, and there is inadequate information to perform a correct analysis.

b. A significant difference was found in one or more baseline characteristics that are known prognostic factors or confounders, but no adjustments were made for this in the analysis.

Minor Flaws

a. The analytical techniques described are incorrect, but there is adequate information to perform a correct analysis.

(continued)

TABLE 1.3   (continued)

b. Means and tests for statistical significance are presented with no measure of the variance.

c. Results are presented in graphical form and tests for significance are presented without giving the actual mean values used to create the graph.

d. Withdrawals are not handled appropriately.

e. Post-hoc subgroup analysis is performed.

f. One-sided tests are inappropriately used for testing statistical significance.

Source: Hadorn, D. C., Baker, D., Hodges, J. S., Hicks, N. (1996). Rating the quality of evidence for clinical practice guidelines. *Journal of Clinical Epidemiology 49, 749–754.*

of the following chapters, MA and other studies cited may be judged by these ways of classifying the quality of evidence.

Use of well-validated and reliable measurement instruments to assess the need for development of SM skills as well as outcomes of intervention intended to achieve them is important but uncommon. Does the instrument consistently yield more or less the same results when administered on several occasions to stable participants, across raters, with the same rater at different times, or with parallel forms of the test (reliability)? Do scores from the instrument relate to other measures in the way one would expect if they are measuring what they are supposed to measure or support hypotheses based on theory (construct validity)? Does an instrument designed to measure change in people over time, including responses to an intervention, detect minimal meaningful differences (responsiveness, also called sensitivity) (Guyatt, Walter, Norman, 1987)?

Internal consistency is a measure of homogeneity of items in a scale, most commonly described by Cronbach's alpha values, with .70–.90 being considered acceptable, and values in the middle .90s necessary for judgments made about individuals. Test-retest reliability should be in the .70–.80 range. Content validity is evaluated logically by consensus of patients and expert opinion, reviews of literature, and assessment of existing instruments. Criterion validity is the correlation between the measure and a gold-standard measure of the same attribute with validity for prediction for groups of people being .60–.70 and predictions for individuals being at least .80 (Redman, 2002).

The number of instruments that directly measure SM is apparently very small. A compendium of related instruments — measures of knowledge, more general SE as opposed to SM SE, and attitudes — may be found in Redman (2003).

Health Policy

Chronic disease affects more than 100 million Americans, with many having more than one condition, and accounts for half of total health care costs. Clearly, policies that support managing these disabilities and their effects are important. Even though cost-effectiveness of SM preparation has been established for some chronic diseases (Gallefoss, Bakke, 2001) and its superiority to alternative methods of chronic disease management such as anticoagulation clinics is well recognized, health care regulatory and payment policy usually does not support SM preparation. For example, diabetes educators have had to wage a decade-long campaign for legislation to mandate coverage for diabetes SM training, equipment, and supplies.

Much health policy is developed by private organizations, including managed care plans, accreditors, and those who purchase care. Several policy tools can be used to build SM preparation into these plans. Explicit coverage of these services as a benefit is important but unlikely to be sufficient without financial rewards to assure that the services are actually delivered. Purchasers can negotiate inclusion of SM preparation into their contractual agreements with providers, including specific targets for improvement of SM and even placing a percentage of the premium at risk for meeting these targets. Currently, few systems are in place to measure receipt of SM preparation services, and it has been difficult to get them added to existing quality measure sets. The most effective combination of incentives and requirements is not clear (Schauffler, 1999).

Disease state management programs encompass appropriate preparation for SM in a broad population-based focus, including undiagnosed individuals at high risk and using an integrated, systematic, and aggressive case management. They include proactive interventions along the continuum of care, with well-designed clinical pathways, visits by highly trained nurses, telephone monitoring and around-the-clock availability, standardized teaching tools, and outcome measurement. Home visits include extensive physical assessment and activity tolerance assessments, instructions on diet, medication review, and risk factor modification. Patients are held accountable for their role in care, and telephone monitoring supplements home visits.

The disease management approach is ideally suited for use in illnesses that are chronic in nature, vary in severity, use extensive health care resources, and can be affected by patients' SM of their symptoms over time. These programs develop knowledge and skills in patients for managing the disease while at the same time remaining a key resource for them. They can produce dramatic improvements in patients' quality of life and decreased costs, particularly through reductions in emergency department (ED) visits and hospitalizations. In one disease management program, the average number of ED visits was reduced by 92% and the average number of hospital admissions fell by 84%. Disease management approaches acknowledge that patients labeled as noncompliant frequently have the desire to be compliant but do not have the knowledge needed to control their disease. Others have treatable depression or anxiety (Hohenleitner, Minniti, 1998).

Many HMOs offer disease management programs for only two or three conditions. A survey of chronic disease management activities found that while essentially all provided patient education to assist patients with SM, most depended on traditional information-oriented resources, with only 18% offering SM support that employed approaches already found to be effective. Those programs that improve patient outcomes share several characteristics:

- They use explicit plans and guidelines based on evidence.
- They reorganize the practice to meet needs of patients requiring more time, a broad array of resources, and closer follow-up.
- They provide systematic attention to the information, behavioral changes, and psychosocial needs of patients.
- They provide ready access to necessary expertise.
- They have supportive information systems.

Evidence suggests that effective disease management programs contributing to SM preparation depend on sustained attention to the SM needs of patients rather than the more typical concentrated dose of didactics at the time of diagnosis with little to follow (Wagner, Davis, Schaefer, Von Korff, Austin, 2001; Wagner, 1997).

A MA of 102 studies found patient education (instructions to patients on how their conditions could be managed, which might be called SM) to be the most commonly used intervention in disease management programs. It was associated with improvements in patient disease control (Weingarten et al., 2002).

For some chronic diseases such as asthma, nationally coordinated coalitions of local organizations have turned improvement in asthma care, including SM preparation, into a movement (Schmidt, Fulwood, Lenfant, 1999).

Current policies that severely limit access to SM preparation most disadvantage those with limited literacy, cognitive ability, or formal education because they do not have skills or contacts to learn SM on their own and often face other barriers associated with poverty.

Summary

Clearly, development of SM preparation effective for and available to the wide range of individuals who need it is a revolution that has been slow in the making. To become reality, this revolution requires a dramatic change in provider attitudes and goals, a stronger research base, consensus about appropriate outcomes, and enactment and testing of policy incentives. The degree to which it will be sustained and advanced is not yet clear. What is clear is its importance to the well-being of patients, their families, and their communities.

References

Atkinson, R. K., Derry, S. J., Renkl, A., Wortham, D. (2000). Learning from examples: Instructional principles from the worked examples research. *Review of Educational Research 70*, 181–214.

Caplin, D. L., Creer, T. L. (2001). A self-management program for adult asthma. III. Maintenance and relapse of skills. *Journal of Asthma 38*, 343–356.

Daly, A., Leontos, C. (1999). Legislation for health care coverage for diabetes self-management training, equipment and supplies: Past, present and future. *Diabetes Spectrum 12*, 222–230.

Devins, G. M., Cameron, J. I., Edworthy, S. M. (2000). Chronic disabling disease. In Radnitz, C. L. (ed). *Cognitive-behavioral therapy for persons with disabilities*. Northvale, NJ: Jason Aronson.

Elliott, T. R., Shewchuk, R. M. (2000). Problem-solving therapy for family caregivers of persons with severe physical disabilities. In Radnitz, C. L. (ed). *Cognitive-behavioral therapy for persons with disabilities*. Northvale, NJ: Jason Aronson.

Elliott, T. R., Shewchuk, R. M., Miller, C. M., Richards, J. S. (2001). Profiles in problem solving: Psychological well-being and distress among persons with diabetes mellitus. *Journal of Clinical Psychology in Medical Settings 8*, 283–291.

Estabrooks, C., et al. (2001). Decision aids: Are they worth it? A systematic review. *Journal of Health Services Research Policy 6*, 170–182.

Ferzacca, S. (2000). "Actually, I don't feel that bad": Managing diabetes and the clinical encounter. *Medical Anthropology Quarterly 14*, 28–50.

Fisher, H. R. (2001). The needs of parents with chronically sick children: A literature review. *Journal of Advanced Nursing 36*, 600–607.

Fox, D. M. (1995). *Power and illness. The failure and future of American health policy*. Sacramento: University of California Press.

Gallefoss, F., Bakke, P. S. (2001). Cost-effectiveness of self-management in asthmatics: A one-year follow-up randomized controlled trial. *European Respiratory Journal 17*, 201–213.

Guyatt, G., Walter, S., Norman, G. (1987). Measuring change over time: Assessing the usefulness of evaluative instruments. *Journal of Chronic Disease 40,* 58–75.

Hadorn, D. C., Baker, D., Hodges, J. S., Hicks, N. (1996). Rating the quality of evidence for clinical practice guidelines. *Journal of Clinical Epidemiology 49,* 749–754.

Hardeman, W., et al. (2002). Application of the theory of planned behaviour in behaviour change interventions: A systematic review. *Psychology and Health 17,* 123–158.

Hohenleitner, S. G., Minniti, M. J. (1998). Developing effective disease state management programs. *Home Health Care Management Practice 10*(4), 11–19.

Jonassen, D. H., Hernandez-Serrano, J. (2002). Case-based reasoning and instructional design: Using stories to support problem solving. *Educational Technology, Research and Development 50,* 65–77.

Jonassen, D. H., Peck, K. L., Wilson, B. G. (1999). *Learning with technology: A constructivist perspective.* Columbus, OH: Merrill.

Kirschner, P. A. (2002). Cognitive load theory: Implications of cognitive load theory on the design of learning. *Learning and Instruction 12,* 1–10.

Lorig, K. (1996). Chronic disease self-management. *American Behavioral Scientist 39,* 676–683.

Lorig, K. R., et al. (1999). Evidence suggesting that a chronic disease self-management program can improve health status while reducing hospitalization. *Medical Care 37,* 5–14.

Lorig, K. R., et al. (2001). Chronic disease self-management program: Two-year health status and health care utilization outcomes. *Medical Care 11,* 1217–1223.

McKay, H. G., King, D., Eaking, E. G., Seeley, J. R., Glasgow, R. E. (2001). The diabetes network Internet-based physical activity intervention. *Diabetes Care 24,* 1328–1334.

Nezu, C. M., et al. (1999). Cancer psychological distress: Two investigations regarding the role of social problem-solving. *Journal of Psychosocial Oncology 16*(3/4), 27–40.

Norris, S. L., Engelgau, M. M., Narayan, K. M. (2001). Effectiveness of self-management training in type 2 diabetes. *Diabetes Care 24,* 561–587.

Partridge, M. R., Hill, S. R. (2002). Enhancing care for people with asthma: The role of communication, education, training and self-management. *European Respiratory Journal 16*, 333–348.

Peeples, M., Mulcahy, K., Tomley, C., Weaver, T. (2001). The conceptual framework of the National Diabetes Education Outcomes System (NDEOS). *The Diabetes Educator 27*, 547–562.

Petrie, K. J., Cameron, L. D., Ellis, C. J., Buick, D., Weinman, J. (2002). Changing illness perceptions after myocardial infarction: An early intervention randomized controlled trial. *Psychosomatic Medicine 64*, 580–586.

Prochaska, J. O., Velicer, W. F. (1997). The transtheoretical model of behavior change. *American Journal of Health Promotion 12*, 38–48.

Redman, B. K. (2001). *The practice of patient education,* 9th ed. St. Louis: Mosby.

Redman, B. K. (2002). *Measurement instruments in clinical ethics.* Thousand Oaks, CA: Sage.

Redman, B. K. (2003). *Measurement tools in patient education,* 2nd ed. New York: Springer Publishing.

Riegel, B., Carlson, B., Glaser, D. (2000). Development and testing of a clinical tool measuring self management of heart failure. *Heart & Lung 29*, 4–12.

Sahler, O. J. A., et al. (2002). Problem-solving skills training for mothers of children with newly diagnosed cancer: A randomized trial. *Developmental and Behavioral Pediatrics 23*(2), 77–86.

Schauffler, H. H. (1999). Policy tools for building health education and preventive counseling into managed care. *American Journal of Preventive Medicine 17*, 309–314.

Schiaffino, K. M., Cea, C. D. (1995). Assessing chronic illness representations: The Implicit Models of Illness Questionnaire. *Journal of Behavioral Medicine 18*, 531–548.

Schmidt, T. K., Fulwood, R., Lenfant, C. (1999). The National Asthma Education and Prevention Program. *Chest 116*, 235S–236S.

Sorenson, S., Pinquart, M., Habil, C., Duberstein, P. (2002). How effective are interventions with caregivers? An updated meta-analysis. *The Gerontologist 42*, 356–372.

Thorne, S. E. (1999). Rethinking the problem of noncompliance in chronic mental illness. In Guimon, J., Fischer, W., Sartorius, N. (eds). *The image of madness: The public facing mental illness and psychiatric treatment.* Basel: Karger.

Thorne, S. E., Nyhlin, K. T., Paterson, B. L. (2000). Attitudes toward patient expertise in chronic illness. *International Journal of Nursing Studies 37,* 303–311.

Thorne, S. E., Paterson, B. L. (2000). Two decades of insider research: What we know and don't know about chronic illness experience. In Fitzpatrick J. J., Goeppinger, J. (eds). *Annual Review of Nursing Research 18,* 3–25.

Van Gerven, P. W. M., Paas, F. G. W. C., Van Meerienboer, J. J. G., Schmidt, H. G. (2002). Cognitive load theory and the acquisition of complex cognitive skills in the elderly: Towards an integrative framework. *Educational Gerontology 26,* 503–521.

Wagner, E. H. (1997). Managed care and chronic illness: Health services research needs. *Health Services Research 32,* 702–714.

Wagner, E. H., Davis, C., Schaefer, J., Von Korff, M., Austin, B. (2001). A survey of leading chronic disease management programs. In Funk, S. G., Tournquist, E. M., Leeman, J., Miles, M. S., Harrell, J. S. (eds). *Key aspects of preventing and managing chronic illness.* New York: Springer Publishing.

Weingarten, S. R., et al. (2002). Interventions used in disease management programmes for patients with chronic illness — which ones work? Meta-analysis of published reports. *British Medical Journal 325,* 925–928.

2
Cancer Self-Management Preparation

Probably because much of the psychosocial work in cancer has focused on coping with the high level of psychological distress and adjustment to a cancer diagnosis, surprisingly few of the elements of preparation for SM are available for persons with cancer and their lay caregivers. These patients need to perform and/or need help in performing disease and treatment monitoring, medication administration, emotional support, and assistance with personal and instrumental care. Because most aspects of cancer curative and palliative care now take place on an outpatient basis, most care occurs at home.

An example of a poorly studied issue accompanying this shift to SM is under- or overadherence to self-administered medication, from a "more is better" approach or confusion about dosage. The dosing schedule is an important factor in the effectiveness of some chemotherapeutic agents, so taking drugs more or less frequently than prescribed may affect therapeutic efficacy. Few studies of cancer patients have evaluated the relationship between adherence level and achievement of the treatment goal (Partridge, Avorn, Wang, Winer, 2002).

Families and their patients with advanced cancer are particularly vulnerable to these shifts in care. These patients are likely to receive aggressive therapy and frequently report considerable numbers of side effects. Alternatively, their care may shift from active treatment with the goal of cure to symptom management with the goal of comfort. To date, the oncology care system has not fully incorporated "family care" for patients at home. In addition, few data are available to define good versus poor outcomes for caregiver care. What are reasonable levels of symptom management? How precisely can family members monitor equipment and changes in critical parameters? Definitions of success are important to caregivers' sense of SE and mastery, and health professionals need to know who does not and cannot provide competent care (Given, Given, Kozachik, 2001).

Despite the fact that the burden and distress on family caregivers has been studied since the early 1980s, few effective strategies to guide family members in caring for patients with advanced cancer have been documented. If family members are competent and supported while delivering care, they will be less anxious and see experiences of patient management in a more positive light (Given, Given, Kozachik, 2001).

Standards for Self-Management Preparation
None could be located.

Effective Interventions and Measurement Instruments
Cognitive problems can occur in both adults and children who experience cranial irradiation, surgery, chemotherapy, and biologic response modifiers. Except in those patients with central nervous system involvement, these cognitive changes are relatively subtle. Patients may report problems with concentration, short-term memory, and problem solving. The typical course of cognitive changes associated with cancer treatment is not known but may well interfere with the learning necessary for SM preparation. A body of intervention research that focuses on dealing with this symptom is lacking (Nail, 2001).

Portions of the full range of intervention strategies identified as important to SM preparation are available in oncology. Most comprehensive is the PRO-SELF program for symptom management among adult patients receiving cancer treatment, which was developed and tested by Dodd and colleagues. This program is designed to provide patients with the information, skills, and support needed to engage effectively and consistently in prescribed self-care symptom management so as to decrease the symptom severity associated with disease and treatment.

Dodd and Miaskowski (2000) note that most symptom management strategies are not evidence-based, are quite variable in terms of the information and skills training that they provide to the patient to monitor and manage anticipated symptoms, and are unclear regarding the desired outcomes. Chemotherapy protocols are becoming more complex and aggressive, causing an increase in treatment-related morbidity. Symptoms are obviously controlled for patient comfort and quality of life, but because uncontrolled symptoms can decrease dosage, they may lead to delays in administering chemotherapy and make patients reluctant to take prescribed therapy. Frequently patients wait until side effects become severe and persistent before initiating self-care measures.

PRO-SELF programs provide self-care exercises for the skills necessary to prevent four major side effects of chemotherapy: nausea, vomiting, mucositis, and infection. Patients become proficient and confident in these skills by performing the skill correctly, consistently, and in a timely manner, and by being able to evaluate whether the prescribed activity is effective. For example, to decrease morbidity associated with chemotherapy-induced mucositis, one group of patients was taught, supervised, and evaluated by return demonstration how and when to care for their mouths. Problems associated with mucositis include pain, local infection, and decreased ability to take food or fluids. Patients learn to care for their mouths while on chemotherapy and to recognize that sores or white spots in the mouth, pain or difficulty in eating or drinking, and unusual amounts of bleeding must be reported to the health professional (Larson and others, 1998).

Each PRO-SELF module includes information and self-care exercises such as a log on which patients record their side effects and SM activities used to manage them. The program also provides equipment such as a thermometer and a flashlight to examine mouths and assistive support by nurses who are available to coach care providers.

The PRO-SELF module for pain control is based on problems that patients experienced in attempting to put a pain management regimen into practice:

- Accessing medication and information
- Tailoring prescribed regimens to meet individual needs
- Managing side effects
- Managing new or unusual pain
- Managing multiple symptoms simultaneously

The module teaches patients how to keep a daily pain diary and how to evaluate the effectiveness of their pain control.

In addition, many cancer patients had difficulty titrating dosages to their own biologic responses, perception of pain, and daily patterns of activity and priorities. Some miscalculated dosages or didn't know how to measure medications. Others couldn't see patterns in, for example, nighttime pain and the need for higher bedtime dosages of their analgesics. Patients with cancer had to manage side effects, most troubling being constipation, causing them to decrease opioid dosage to an ineffective level. For reasons that are not fully understood, some patients continued to have difficulty adhering to pain management regimens even after intensive educational interventions, and virtually no research attention has been paid to the process of pain management by patients and their family caregivers (Schumacher and others, 2002).

Even as patients found effective approaches, the nature of their pain would change as a result of disease progression or response to treatment, leaving them uncertain about what was happening and unclear about how to change their behavior. Patients had difficulty managing multiple symptoms simultaneously — pain, hot flashes, and sleeplessness as a result of cancer treatment and bone metastasis; symptoms from other concurrent chronic illnesses; and side effects from the array of medications prescribed for all of their diseases. Clearly, some patients had difficulty with memory or thinking analytically and processing complex information, which affected their problem-solving abilities. Provision of information to these patients and their families was insufficient to provide pain control in the home setting; nurse coaching related to ongoing problem solving continued for some time. Rather than demanding strict adherence to a standardized regimen, pain management requires ongoing problem solving with adjustment and modifications to meet patients' needs (Schumacher et al., 2002).

Closely related to this issue is Mishel et al.'s (2002) work on uncertainty management intervention delivered weekly for an eight-week period by phone for men with localized prostate cancer. *Uncertainty* is the inability to determine the meaning of illness-related events, when patients lack the information or knowledge needed to fully understand their illness, treatment, and treatment residuals. Patients with prostate carcinoma have reported they do not receive adequate help for the problems that result from the disease or its treatment. Such a deficit can hamper decision making and inhibit performance of problem-oriented coping. Uncertainty management involves promoting cognitive reframing, problem solving, and skills training.

Self-efficacy, the belief that one has mastery over events and can meet challenges as they occur, can be learned. Without intervention, cancer patients' SM SE and adjustment decrease over time, suggesting that interventions given to patients with cancer in the early months following diagnosis may be effective. To increase SM SE, health professionals can take the following steps (Lev et al., 2001):

- Contract with patients to practice specific self-care behaviors (performance accomplishments)
- Have patients view videotape of previous cancer patients who dealt successfully with diagnosis and treatment care (vicarious experience)
- Provide verbal encouragement and assert that the patient has the ability to provide self-care (verbal persuasion)
- Provide realistic symptom interpretation and maintain a calm attitude (physiological state)

In Lev et al.'s RCT, the researchers tested the SE-enhancing intervention and found that at four to eight months after women began chemotherapy for breast cancer, members of the experimental group had a better quality of life and less symptom distress than did members of the control group.

Problem-solving therapy has been used in several studies. Cancer patients characterized by less effective problem-solving ability were found to report higher levels of depression and anxiety as well as a greater number of cancer-related problems (Nezu, Nezu, Friedman, Houts, Faddis, 1997). A RCT of problem-solving therapy in home care training for women younger than 50 years of age with breast cancer helped those with average or good problem-solving skills to decrease stressors and solve problems associated with diagnosis, treatment, physical side effects, and psychological problems of cancer but was not effective for those with poor problem-solving skills. The intervention involved reviewing problem-solving techniques and resolving sample problems using worksheets specifically designed for a step-by-step approach (Allen et al., 2002).

The two measures relevant to SM preparation for patients with cancer that were located tested SE. The Cancer Behavior Inventory (CBI) is a measure of SE for coping with cancer, which includes many SM behaviors. It has two forms: a 33-item long form (CBI-L) and a 14-item brief form (CBI-B; alpha, .85). Factors for the long version and scoring for both versions may be found in Figure 2.1; Figures 2.2 and 2.3 represent the CBI instruments. Scores are obtained by summing across all items. Psychosocial adjustment and quality of life are highly correlated with most factors on the CBI-L, supporting its validity. Test-retest reliability at one week was .74 (Merluzzi, Martinez, 1997). Note that the CBI is focused more on coping SE than on SE for SM skills.

Lev and others (2001) used a SE instrument specific to self-care but not specific to cancer, called Strategies Used by Patients to Promote Health (SUPPH). Internal consistency reliability was in the range .94–.96, with test-retest reliability of .94. Positive correlation with measures of values about health behavior management supported convergent validation (Lev,

---

CBI-L (Version 2.0)

The CBI is scored by summing the patients' ratings across all 33 items to obtain an overall score (Cronbach's α = .94). Given the factor structure of the CBI, it can also be scored by factor.

Factor 1: Maintenance of activity and independence (α = .86)
Sum of 5 items: 1, 4, 8, 21, 30

Factor 2: Seeking and understanding medical information (α = .88)
Sum of 5 items: 15, 5, 9, 19, 29

Factor 3: Stress management for medical appointments
Sum of 5 items: 6, 12, 17, 23, 27

Factor 4: Coping with treatment-related side effects (α = .82)
Sum of 5 items: 10, 13, 25, 31, 32

Factor 5: Accepting cancer/maintaining a positive attitude (α = .86)
Sum of 5 items: 2, 3, 24, 28, 33

Factor 6: Affective regulation (α = .81)
Sum of 5 items: 11, 14, 18, 20, 22

Factor 7: Seeking support (α = .80)
Sum of 3 items: 7, 16, 26

For comparison of means across scales (factors), you would divide the summed score by the number of items in the scale.

CBI-B (Version 2.0)

The scoring for Form B is simply the sum of the 14 items (α = .85).

Source: Thomas V. Merluzzi.

FIGURE 2.1 Factors and scoring for the Cancer Behavior Inventory (CBI)

Paul, Owen, 1999). As may be seen in Figure 2.4, the respondent is asked to rate the degree of confidence he or she has in carrying out specific self-care behaviors. SUPPH is scored by summing reponses, with scores ranging from 36 to 180.

Cancer Behavior Inventory, Long Form (CBI-L)

This questionnaire contains many things that a person might do when receiving treatment for cancer. We are interested in your judgment of how confident you are that you can accomplish those things. Make sure your ratings accurately reflect your *confidence whether or not* you have done it in the past. Your ratings reflect *your confidence* that you can do these things now (or in the near future).

Please read each numbered item. Then rate that item on how confident you are that you can accomplish that behavior. Circle a number on the scale. If you circle a "1," you would be stating that you are not at all confident that you can accomplish that behavior. If you circle a "9," you would be stating that you are totally confident that you can accomplish that behavior. Numbers in the middle of the scale indicate that you are moderately confident that you can accomplish that behavior.

Please rate *all* items. If you are not sure about an item please rate it as best you can.

	NOT AT ALL CONFIDENT				MODERATELY CONFIDENT				TOTALLY CONFIDENT
1. Maintaining independence	1	2	3	4	5	6	7	8	9
2. Maintaining a positive attitude	1	2	3	4	5	6	7	8	9
3. Accepting that I have cancer	1	2	3	4	5	6	7	8	9
4. Maintaining work activity	1	2	3	4	5	6	7	8	9
5. Asking nurses questions	1	2	3	4	5	6	7	8	9
6. Remaining relaxed throughout treatments and not allowing scary thoughts to upset me	1	2	3	4	5	6	7	8	9
7. Seeking support from people and groups outside the family	1	2	3	4	5	6	7	8	9
8. Maintaining a daily routine	1	2	3	4	5	6	7	8	9
9. Asking technologists questions	1	2	3	4	5	6	7	8	9
10. Coping with hair loss	1	2	3	4	5	6	7	8	9
11. Using denial	1	2	3	4	5	6	7	8	9
12. Remaining relaxed throughout treatment (chemotherapy, radiation)	1	2	3	4	5	6	7	8	9
13. Coping with physical changes	1	2	3	4	5	6	7	8	9
14. Ignoring things that cannot be dealt with	1	2	3	4	5	6	7	8	9
15. Actively participating in treatment decisions	1	2	3	4	5	6	7	8	9
16. Sharing feelings of concern	1	2	3	4	5	6	7	8	9

FIGURE 2.2

		NOT AT ALL CONFIDENT				MODERATELY CONFIDENT				TOTALLY CONFIDENT
17.	Remaining relaxed while waiting at least one hour for my appointment	1	2	3	4	5	6	7	8	9
18.	Expressing personal feelings of anger or hostility	1	2	3	4	5	6	7	8	9
19.	Seeking information about cancer or cancer treatments	1	2	3	4	5	6	7	8	9
20.	Expressing negative feelings about cancer	1	2	3	4	5	6	7	8	9
21.	Keeping busy with activities	1	2	3	4	5	6	7	8	9
22.	Finding an escape	1	2	3	4	5	6	7	8	9
23.	Reducing any anxiety associated with getting my blood drawn	1	2	3	4	5	6	7	8	9
24.	Maintaining a sense of humor	1	2	3	4	5	6	7	8	9
25.	Accepting physical changes or limitations caused by cancer treatment	1	2	3	4	5	6	7	8	9
26.	Seeking consolation	1	2	3	4	5	6	7	8	9
27.	Reducing any nausea associated with treatment (chemotherapy, radiation)	1	2	3	4	5	6	7	8	9
28.	Maintaining hope	1	2	3	4	5	6	7	8	9
29.	Asking physicians questions	1	2	3	4	5	6	7	8	9
30.	Doing something, anything	1	2	3	4	5	6	7	8	9
31.	Managing pain	1	2	3	4	5	6	7	8	9
32.	Managing nausea and vomiting	1	2	3	4	5	6	7	8	9
33.	Controlling my negative feelings about cancer	1	2	3	4	5	6	7	8	9

Sources: Merluzzi, Thomas V., Nairn, Raymond C., Sanchez, Mary Ann Martinez.

FIGURE 2.2 *(continued)*

CANCER BEHAVIOR INVENTORY, BRIEF FORM (CBI-B)

This questionnaire contains many things that a person might do when receiving treatment for cancer. We are interested in your judgment of how confident you are that you can accomplish those things. Make sure your ratings accurately reflect your *confidence whether or not* you have done it in the past. Your ratings reflect *your confidence* that you can do these things now (or in the near future).

Please read each numbered item. Then rate that item on how confident you are that you can accomplish that behavior. Circle a number on the scale. If you circle a "1," you would be stating that you are not at all confident that you can accomplish that behavior. If you circle a "9," you would be stating that you are totally confident that you can accomplish that behavior. Numbers in the middle of the scale indicate that you are moderately confident that you can accomplish that behavior.

Please rate *all* items. If you are not sure about an item please rate it as best you can.

	NOT AT ALL CONFIDENT				MODERATELY CONFIDENT				TOTALLY CONFIDENT
1. Maintaining independence	1	2	3	4	5	6	7	8	9
2. Maintaining a positive attitude	1	2	3	4	5	6	7	8	9
3. Maintaining a sense of humor	1	2	3	4	5	6	7	8	9
4. Expressing negative feelings about cancer	1	2	3	4	5	6	7	8	9
5. Using denial	1	2	3	4	5	6	7	8	9
6. Maintaining work activity	1	2	3	4	5	6	7	8	9
7. Remaining relaxed throughout treatments and not allowing scary thoughts to upset me	1	2	3	4	5	6	7	8	9
8. Actively participating in treatment decisions	1	2	3	4	5	6	7	8	9
9. Asking physicians questions	1	2	3	4	5	6	7	8	9
10. Seeking consolation	1	2	3	4	5	6	7	8	9
11. Sharing feelings of concern	1	2	3	4	5	6	7	8	9
12. Managing nausea and vomiting	1	2	3	4	5	6	7	8	9
13. Coping with physical changes	1	2	3	4	5	6	7	8	9
14. Remaining relaxed while waiting at least one hour for my appointment	1	2	3	4	5	6	7	8	9

Sources: Merluzzi, Thomas V., Nairn, Raymond C., Sanchez, Mary Ann Martinez.

FIGURE 2.3

ID SUPPH-29

Your answers on this questionnaire will help us to learn more about how people deal with illness. Some people use their own methods such as prayer, relaxation techniques, visualization, physical exercise, and other techniques which they feel are helpful. We are interested in what you do. There are no right or wrong answers to these questions. Your responses are strictly anonymous.

Below is a list of behaviors. How much **confidence** do you have in doing these behaviors? Rate your confidence.

	VERY LITTLE	CONFIDENCE			QUITE A LOT
1. Excluding upsetting thoughts from my consciousness	1	2	3	4	5
2. Using relaxation techniques to decrease my anxiety	1	2	3	4	5
3. Finding ways of alleviating my stress	1	2	3	4	5
4. Using a specific technique to manage my stress	1	2	3	4	5
5. Doing things that helped me to cope with previous emotional difficulties	1	2	3	4	5
6. Practicing stress reduction techniques even when I'm feeling sick	1	2	3	4	5
7. Managing to keep anxiety about illness from becoming overwhelming	1	2	3	4	5
8. Thinking of myself as better off than people who became ill when they were younger than I am now	1	2	3	4	5
9. Focusing on something not associated with my illness as a way of decreasing my anxiety	1	2	3	4	5
10. Believing that using a technique to manage treatment stress will actually work	1	2	3	4	5
11. Choosing among treatment alternatives recommended by my physician the one that seems right for me	1	2	3	4	5
12. Making my own decision regarding treatment alternatives	1	2	3	4	5
13. Deciding for myself whether or not to have treatment	1	2	3	4	5i
14. Experiencing life's pleasures since I became ill	1	2	3	4	5

FIGURE 2.4

		Very Little		Confidence		Quite A Lot
15.	Doing special things for myself to make life better	1	2	3	4	5
16.	Convincing myself I can manage the treatment stress	1	2	3	4	5
17.	Helping other people going through illness and treatment	1	2	3	4	5
18.	Convincing myself the treatment is not so bad	1	2	3	4	5
19.	Keeping my stress within healthy limits	1	2	3	4	5
20.	Appreciating what is really important in life	1	2	3	4	5
21.	Believing I can find strength within myself for healing	1	2	3	4	5
22.	Convincing myself I'll be O.K.	1	2	3	4	5
23.	Finding a way to help me get through this time	1	2	3	4	5
24.	Believing that I really have a positive attitude about my state of health	1	2	3	4	5
25.	Doing things that helped me to cope with previous physical difficulties	1	2	3	4	5
26.	Doing things to control my fatigue	1	2	3	4	5
27.	Finding ways of helping myself feel better if I am feeling blue	1	2	3	4	5
28.	Managing the side effects of treatment so that I can do things I enjoy doing	1	2	3	4	5
29.	Dealing with the frustration of illness and treatment	1	2	3	4	5

Instructions:

The SUPPH-29 is a concise self-report scale. However, a short introduction and period of instruction are needed for the measurement program to be valid. The following introduction was given by research assistants prior to subjects' completion of the scale and was used to introduce the scale verbally to respondents. The individual who introduces the scale needs to stress that the respondents should answer the questions based on their confidence in carrying out the behaviors that follow. Examples of introductions to the scale given by research assistants follow.

People use different ways to adapt to their illness. Some people tell me they use prayer as a way of managing their illness. Other people use relaxation techniques or imagery, where they imagine being in a pleasant place, like

FIGURE 2.4 (continued)

at the mountains or at the beach. Some use physical exercise as a way to adapt. Some people tell me they talk to themselves, saying things like, "Keep on going," "Take one day at a time," or "Be determined." What do you use to help you adapt?

People use different ways to adapt to their illness. Some people tell me they use prayer and some might use relaxation techniques or imagery, where they imagine being in a pleasant place, like at the mountains or at the beach. Others use physical exercise as a way to adapt. Some people tell me they talk to themselves, saying things like, "Keep on going," "Take one day at a time," or "Be determined." What do you use to help you adapt?

If the patient is unable to identify anything, ask whether he or she had anything in the past that was similar, and what the person did at that time. Often while one continues talking to the patient repression strategies, such as reading and watching TV, are identified. Then the questionnaire is begun by incorporating the strategies stated by the patient. For example, "You told me you find it helpful to use relaxation exercises. Think of that as your 'strategy' for dealing with your illness."

Scoring

Scoring the scale involves summing the responses. The description of the 4 factors on the scale follow.

Factor structure of SUPPH-29

Factor	Items	Alpha Estimate
Coping	1, 7, 8, 9, 16, 18, 19, 20, 21, 22, 23, 24, 25, 26, 27, 28, 29	.92
Stress Reduction	2, 3, 4, 5, 6, 10	.86
Making Decisions	.11, 12, 13	.83
Enjoying Life	14, 15, 17	.76

	Coping	Stress	Decisions	Enjoying
Correlations among factors in ESRD subjects				
Coping	. . . . .	.65	.36	.69
Stress Reduction		. . . . .	.47	.52
Making Decisions			. . . . .	.35
Enjoying Life				. . . . .
Correlations among factors in oncology subjects				
Coping	. . . . .	.51	.48	.59
Stress Reduction		. . . . .	.21	.45
Making Decisions			. . . . .	.51
Enjoying Life				. . . . .

FIGURE 2.4 (continued)

Description of Items and Factor Loading

Item	Loading
Factor 1: Coping	
19. Keeping my stress within healthy limits	.76
22. Convincing myself I'll be OK	.73
23. Finding a way to help me get through this time	.71
16. Convincing myself I can manage the treatment stress	.70
29. Dealing with the frustration of illness and treatment	.70
27. Finding ways of helping myself feel better if I am feeling blue	.64
18. Convincing myself the treatment is not so bad	.62
24. Believing that I really have a positive attitude about my state of health	.59
21. Believing I can find strength within myself for healing	.58
7. Managing to keep anxiety about treatment from becoming overwhelming	.53
8. Thinking of myself as better off than people who became ill when they were younger than I am now	.50
28. Managing the side effects of treatment so that I can do things I enjoy doing	.48
1. Excluding upsetting thoughts from my consciousness	.48
9. Focusing on something not associated with my treatment as a way of decreasing my anxiety	.45
25. Doing things that helped me to cope with previous physical difficulties	.44
20. Appreciating what is really important in life	.41
26. Doing things to control my fatigue	.40
Factor 2: Stress Reduction	
6. Practicing stress reduction techniques even when I'm feeling sick	.81
10. Believing that using a technique to manage treatment stress will actually work	.75
2. Using relaxation techniques to decrease my anxiety	.73
3. Finding ways of alleviating my stress	.69
4. Using a specific technique to manage my stress	.65
5. Doing things that helped me to cope with previous emotional difficulties	.54

FIGURE 2.4 (continued)

Item	Loading
Factor 3: Making Decisions	
12. Making my own decision regarding treatment alternatives	.87
13. Deciding for myself whether or not to have treatment	.76
11. Choosing among treatment alternatives recommended by my physician the one that seems right for me	.74
Factor 4: Enjoying Life	
14. Experiencing life's pleasures since I became ill	.62
15. Doing special things for myself to make life better	.61
17. Helping other people going through cancer treatment	.47

Sources: Lev, E. L., Daley, K., Conner, N., Reith, M., Fernandez, C., & Owen, S. V. (2001). An intervention to increase quality of life and self-care self-efficacy and decrease symptoms in breast cancer patients. *Scholarly Inquiry for Nursing Practice: An International Journal* 15(3), 277–294; Lev, E. L., Paul, D. B., & Owen, S. V. (1999). Age, self-efficacy, and change in patients' adjustment to cancer. *Cancer Practice* 7(4), 170–176; Lev, E. L., & Owen, S. V. (1998). A prospective study of adjustment to hemodialysis. *American Nephrology Nurses' Association Journal* 25(5), 495–506; Lev, E. L., & Owen, S. V. (1996). A measure of self-care self-efficacy. *Research in Nursing & Health 19,* 421–429. Reproduced by permission of Elise Lev.

FIGURE 2.4   *(continued)*

Management by Family Caregivers

As the locus of cancer care continues to shift from the hospital to the home, increasing numbers of patients are being cared for by family members. With shorter lengths of stay in the acute care setting, cancer patients are returning home with complex care needs that require a high degree of skill (Barg et al., 1998). These needs include symptom management, monitoring for changes in hallmark symptoms, recognizing when symptoms appear out of control or current measures are ineffective, equipment care (e.g., infusion pumps or IVs), and patient transport and advocacy (Given, Given, Kozachik, 2001).

Interventions for family members related to problem SM for persons with cancer has been of concern. Table 2.1 provides a

Table 2.1   Indicators of Skill in Family Caregiving Processes

Monitoring

1. Uses appropriate specificity
2. Notices subtle changes
3. Notices verbal and nonverbal indicators of care receiver well-being
4. Uses instruments for monitoring when appropriate
5. Uses appropriate vigilance
6. Makes accurate observations
7. Keeps a written record when appropriate
8. Notices patterns

Interpreting

1. Recognizes deviations from normal or expected clinical course
2. Recognizes that something is "different" or "wrong"
3. Judges seriousness of a problem
4. Seeks explanations for unexplained signs and symptoms
5. Asks detailed questions for the purpose of developing an explanation
6. Makes correct attributions
7. Uses a reference point in making sense of observations
8. Considers multiple explanations for an observation

Making decisions

1. Takes into account multiple illness care demands
2. Weighs competing illness care demands
3. Weighs the importance of conflicting priorities
4. Attends to multiple care issues at once
5. Thinks ahead about possible consequences of a given action

(continued)

Table 2.1 (continued)

Taking action

1. Recurring actions are taken at effective intervals
2. Uses effective "reminders" to time actions
3. Paces actions to correspond with ill person's pace
4. Times actions with respect to the rhythm of ill person's responses to chemotherapy
5. Times actions with respect to ill person's daily rhythm of responses
6. Times intermittent or one-time actions appropriately
7. Takes own needs into account in timing actions
8. Organizes multiple actions systematically
9. Develops routines to manage complex tasks
10. Organizes illness care tasks so that ill person can be involved if appropriate
11. Uses a system for remembering when actions are due
12. Uses different tracking systems for scheduled actions and actions that are taken as needed
13. Has the ability to take action on multiple issues at once

Making adjustments

1. Adjusts amount of food, PRN medications, rest, exercise, and so forth, until optimum comfort and symptom management achieved
2. Modifies long-standing routines to accommodate illness situation
3. Modifies environment to accommodate illness situation
4. Tries multiple strategies until a solution to caregiving problems found
5. Uses "mistakes" as an opportunity for learning
6. Considers what led up to a "mistake" and alters what appears to be the source of the problem
7. Searches for an alternative when one illness care strategy no longer works
8. Uses creativity in problem solving

(continued)

Table 2.1 (continued)

Accessing resources

1. Seeks resources wisely; casts a broad net
2. Uses advice judiciously
3. Seeks authoritative resources when appropriate
4. Weeds out erroneous, inaccurate, or inadequate advice
5. Persists in obtaining resources until what is really needed is found
6. Takes initiative in seeking resources
7. Figures out which health care providers are most accessible, helpful, and knowledgeable
8. Makes own needs known

Source: Schumacher, K. L., Stewart, B. J., Archbold, P. G., Dodd, M. J., Dibble, S. L. (2000). Family caregiving skill: Development of the concept. *Research in Nursing and Health 23*, 191–203. Reprinted by permission of John Wiley & Sons, Inc.

set of indicators of skill for family caregiving processes used in a study of patients receiving chemotherapy for cancer and their primary family caregivers (Schumacher, Stewart, Archbold, Dodd, Dibble, 2000). Barg and colleagues (1998) note that caregivers especially need management preparation at transition points in the patient's course of illness: diagnosis; initiation or cessation of treatment; recurrence; change in treatment goals such as change from curative to palliative treatment; and so on.

The authors found that 65% of the caregivers participating in a psychoeducational intervention reported problems ranging from difficulty to extreme difficulty with watching the patient become more ill and not knowing what to do. Feelings of inadequacy and helplessness arise from the ambiguity inherent in this situation. Seventy-four percent of the sample had significant concerns about their ability to handle the patients' care in the future. The indicators in Table 2.1 provide a way to pinpoint areas in which caregivers are having difficulty, thereby facilitating targeted intervention (Barg et al., 1998).

When caregiving difficulties occur, they often have negative effects on caregivers and care receivers alike, leading to suboptimal symptom and side-effect management, emergency hospitalization and/or unscheduled physician visits, delayed treatment, safety risks, emotional distress for both individuals, and conflict about illness management. The investigators' results suggest that brief periods of nursing instruction may not be sufficient for the development of caregiving skill; rather, ongoing coaching for skill development may be required. In the United States, limited access to professional nurses raises serious concerns about whether family caregivers can get the coaching they need (Schumacher, Stewart, Archbold, Dodd, Dibble, 2000).

References

Allen, S. M., et al. (2002). A problem-solving approach to stress reduction among younger women with breast carcinoma. *Cancer 94,* 3089–3100.

Barg, F. K., et al. (1998). A description of a psychoeducational intervention for family caregivers of cancer patients. *Journal of Family Nursing 4,* 394–411.

Dodd, M. J., Miaskowski, C. (2000). The PRO-SELF program: A self-care intervention program for patients receiving cancer treatment. *Seminars in Oncology Nursing 16,* 300–308.

Given, B. A., Given, C. W., Kozachik, S. (2001). Family support in advanced cancer. *CA 51,* 213–231.

Larson, P. J., et al. (1998). The PRO-SELF Mouth Aware program: An effective approach for reducing chemotherapy-induced mucositis. *Cancer Nursing 21,* 263–268.

Lev, E. L., et al. (2001). An intervention to increase quality of life and self-care self-efficacy and decrease symptoms in breast cancer patients. *Scholarly Inquiry for Nursing Practice 15,* 277–293.

Lev, E. L., Paul, D., Owen, S. V. (1999). Age, self-efficacy and change in patients' adjustment to cancer. *Cancer Practice 7,* 170–176.

Merluzzi, T. V., Martinez, C. S. (1997). Assessment of self-efficacy and coping with cancer: Development and validation of the Cancer Behavioral Inventory. *Health Psychology 16,* 163–170.

Mishel, M. H., et al. (2002). Helping patients with localized prostate carcinoma manage uncertainty and treatment side effects. *Cancer 94,* 1854–1866.

Nail, L. M. (2001). Long-term persistence of symptoms. *Seminars in Oncology Nursing 17,* 249–254.

Nezu, A. M., Nezu, C. M., Friedman, S. H., Houts, P. S., Faddis, S. (1997). Project Genesis: Application of problem-solving therapy to individuals with cancer. *The Behavioral Therapist 20,* 155–158.

Partridge, A. H., Avorn, J., Wang, P. S., Winer, E. P. (2002). Adherence to therapy with oral antineoplastic agents. *Journal of the National Cancer Institute 94,* 652–661.

Schumacher, K. L., et al. (2002). Putting cancer pain management regimens into practice at home. *Journal of Pain and Symptom Management 23,* 369–382.

Schumacher, K. L., Stewart, B. J., Archbold, P. G., Dodd, M. J., Dibble, S. L. (2000). Family caregiving skill: Development of the concept. *Research in Nursing and Health 23,* 191–203.

3

Arthritis Self-Management Preparation

Arthritis is one of the most common chronic conditions, with prevalence rates predicted to increase as the population ages. The largest single cause of disability, it has an unpredictable course, uncertain prognosis, and significant psychosocial impact. Osteoarthritis affects as many as 65% of older adults, and rheumatoid arthritis afflicts about 5% of the general population. Psychological factors are more strongly associated with disability than are disease parameters. Therapies that can prevent or slow organ damage, if they are instituted early, are now available.

Arthritis SM has one dominant well-established model with known outcomes, based on social learning theory, which has been tested in several countries (Arthritis SM Program, ASMP). Several other models of arthritis SM exist and incorporate theoretically important elements. However, actual delivery of these services is believed to be rare in primary care and only slightly more common in the practice of rheumatologists (Mazzuca et al., 1997).

Sufficient research has been done on the effects of patient education in rheumatoid arthritis to warrant a Cochrane review of RCTs (Riemsma, Kirwan, Taal, Rasker, 2002). The intervention in many of the studies in the review goes beyond information-based patient education and contains the elements of SM preparation. The summary of 24 studies found significant effects at first follow-up for scores on disability, joint counts, patient global assessment, and psychological states. In addition, enough studies involving osteoarthritis and rheumatoid arthritis have been carried out to show that SM programs can ameliorate pain and depression. Studies have revealed that training in SM can be beneficial in patients who have moderate to high levels of pain and disability (Keefe et al., 2000). Most measures are outcomes for the disease, not specifically for SM preparation.

Standards for Self-Management Preparation

Standards for arthritis patient education (not limited to SM preparation) are process standards that define adequate needs assessment, planning, curriculum, instructor, and evaluation standards (Burckhardt, 1994). They do not reflect outcomes or set benchmarks.

Effective Interventions and Measurement Instruments

The ASMP strongly emphasizes development of SE with some problem-solving focus but less explicit focus on illness representation models for disease or on stages of change. It is taught two hours per week for six weeks to a group of about 15 participants, in a community setting such as a senior center, library, church, or shopping center. Content includes pathophysiology, medications, personal exercise, pain management, nutrition, appropriate use of joints, communication with providers, and resolution of problems that arise from the illness.

Randomized trials have shown that ASMP increases SE, SM behaviors, exercise, and use of cognitive pain management techniques to decrease pain, and it decreases ambulatory visits to physicians. Longitudinal cohort studies have demonstrated that these effects continue without formal reinforcement for as long as four years. Skills mastery is aided by contracting for SM behavior. A recent study of a three-week version of the ASMP has found that it is not as effective as is the six-week version (Lorig et al., 1998). Leaders teaching ASMP are individuals with arthritis, serving as models. These individuals receive 18 hours of training and follow a detailed protocol of instruction.

Studies of program participants have found that improved outcomes correlate most strongly with a person's level and growth of perceived SE in coping with the consequences of chronic arthritis. At least one study has found no significant clinical benefits from ASMP in the context of primary care physicians' practices. The authors of this study suggest a potential reason for these findings: The populations on which ASMP was originally validated were recruited from larger populations on a voluntary basis and were perhaps ready for change, as opposed to those patients seeing physicians in a primary care practice (Solomon et al., 2002).

This course is currently available in all 50 states and a number of foreign countries (Kruger, Helmick, Callahan, Haddix, 1998). ASMP has been most frequently studied in middle-aged or elderly Caucasian females with at least a twelfth-grade education (Edworthy, 2000). Each year this program reaches 12,000 adults who have been diagnosed with a form of chronic arthritis; for a cohort of 10,000 individuals, it is estimated to save $2.5 million over five years. Its effect on pain reduction is substantial, amounting to an estimated 20% to 30% of, and additive to, that seen with medical interventions such as use of NSAIDs (Kruger, Helmick, Callahan, Haddix, 1998).

Implementing a program such as ASMP requires considerable planning and effort, including sponsorship of an organization affiliated with the community as well as with volunteerism. Individuals from the community must be found and trained to be program leaders, and the pool of leaders needs to be replenished as more courses are given. There is now a great deal of experience with lay-led community SM programs. In addition, some evidence, albeit not from a controlled trial, indicates that training to become a lay leader and conducting an ASMP is associated with improvements in physical and psychological status, arthritis SE, and use of SM techniques for oneself (Edworthy, 2000; Hainsworth, Barlow, 2001).

ASMP is merely one type of SM program and differs in approach from many other such programs, which are typically led by health professionals in hospital settings with patients who have been recruited through clinics. SM preparation intervention programs may include disease information and cognitive pain management skills; exercise; training in activities of daily living; teaching of problem-solving skills, social skills and relaxation training; counseling and therapy biofeedback; and social support. The number of sessions within each program varies enormously, from a single session to 12 or more, with each lasting as little as 20 minutes to 2 hours or more. Telephone contact or self-instruction with a computer program or a manual are used as well.

The components of SM preparation intervention that are most effective are not well understood. In general, cognitive approaches such as modulation of ways of thinking about arthritis are fairly successful in decreasing pain but show few effects on disability (Newman, Mulligan, Steed, 2001). Because the discomfort of the disease fluctuates over time, it is particularly important for studies of effects to include a control group.

Scholten and colleagues (1999) describe a RCT with multiple theoretically potent intervention elements. This program includes content in pathogenesis of rheumatoid arthritis, drug therapy, physiotherapy, practical exercise in remedial gymnastics, use of joint protection devices, psychological counseling, dietetics information about unproved cures, and social assistance. Interactive discussion, problem solving including possible solutions, and goal setting were used to deliver content and achieve goals.

Briefer interventions have also shown positive effects. A controlled trial of osteoarthritis knee self-care education as an adjunct to primary care for inner-city patients achieved notable preservation of function and control of resting knee pain over the subsequent year, compared with attention control. This intervention lasted 30 to 60 minutes and included quadriceps strengthening exercises, control of joint pain and thermal modalities, joint protection, and a problem-solving exercise to develop a plan for maintaining a threatened activity in ways that minimized stress on the knee. Five- to ten-minute phone calls at one week and one month after initial instruction were used as maintenance. The intervention is meant to be an exportable adjunct to primary care. Observed effects were of a magnitude similar to the more labor-intensive and time-consuming ASMP, and 80% of the cost of delivering this self-care education was offset in a year by decreased costs of primary care visits (Mazzuca et al., 1997; Mazzuca, Brandt, Katz, Hanna, Melfi, 1999).

A similar problem-based program (Lindroth et al., 1997) for rheumatoid arthritis involved practice of exercise and joint protection, including use of kitchen tools, and solving of group members' problems. It produced decreases in disability and pain in comparison with a control group.

Other theoretical models might be expected to be effective. Arthritis patients vary considerably in their involvement in SM efforts. Using the transtheoretical model, Keefe and others (2000) found 44% of their sample of arthritis patients to be in precontemplation stage, suggesting they may be resistant to SM. Eleven percent were in the contemplation stage and intending to take action in the future, 22% were in the preparation stage both thinking about change and making some overt behavior changes, and 17% were in the prepared maintenance stage. Consistent with what theory would predict, individuals in the action stage had the highest SE of any of the subgroups. Disease duration was not related to stage.

It is not yet usual to answer the question about which intervention component is effective on which outcome variable and in which patients. For example, some evidence shows that modulation of ways of thinking about arthritis were fairly successful in decreasing pain but had few effects on disability (Newman, Mulligan, Steed, 2001).

Onset of rheumatic disease presents a person with an array of confusing and serious symptoms that are difficult to understand, frequently followed by repeated unsuccessful attempts to cope with the illness. While an intervention focused on illness representations, coping behaviors, and appraisals based on self-regulatory theory might be expected to be successful, little intervention work based on this model has been done (Pimm, 1997).

Two instruments measuring SE are available for assessment of patient need to learn and to measure outcomes of SM preparation. SE appears to be particularly important for patients

Arthritis Self-Efficacy Scale*

Self-Efficacy Pain Subscale

In the following questions, we'd like to know how your arthritis pain affects you. For each of the following questions, please circle the number that corresponds to your level of certainty that you can now perform the following tasks.

1. How certain are you that you can decrease your pain quite a bit?
2. How certain are you that you can continue most of your daily activities?
3. How certain are you that you can keep arthritis pain from interfering with your sleep?
4. How certain are you that you can make a small-to-moderate reduction in your arthritis pain by using methods other than taking extra medication?
5. How certain are you that you can make a large reduction in your arthritis pain by using methods other than taking extra medication?

Self-Efficacy Function Subscale*

We would like to know how confident you are in performing certain daily activities. For each of the following questions, please circle the number that corresponds to your certainty that you can perform the tasks as of now without assistive devices or help from another person. Please consider what you routinely can do, not what would require a single extraordinary effort.

AS OF NOW, HOW CERTAIN ARE YOU THAT YOU CAN:

1. Walk 100 feet on flat ground in 20 seconds?
2. Walk 10 steps downstairs in 7 seconds?
3. Get out of an armless chair quickly, without using your hands for support?
4. Button and unbutton 3 medium-size buttons in a row in 12 seconds?
5. Cut 2 bite-size pieces of meat with a knife and fork in 8 seconds?
6. Turn an outdoor faucet all the way on and all the way off?

7. Scratch your upper back with both your right and left hands?
8. Get in and out of the passenger side of a car without assistance from another person and without physical aids?
9. Put on a long-sleeve front-opening shirt or blouse (without buttoning) in 8 seconds?

Self-Efficacy Other Symptoms Subscale*

In the following questions, we'd like to know how you feel about your ability to control your arthritis. For each of the following questions, please circle the number that corresponds to your level of certainty that you can now perform the following activities or tasks.

1. How certain are you that you can control your fatigue?
2. How certain are you that you can regulate your activity so as to be active without aggravating your arthritis?
3. How certain are you that you can do something to help yourself feel better if you are feeling blue?
4. As compared with other people with arthritis like yours, how certain are you that you can manage arthritis pain during your daily activities?
5. How certain are you that you can manage your arthritis symptoms so that you can do the things you enjoy doing?
6. How certain are you that you can deal with the frustration of arthritis?

---

*Each question is followed by the scale:

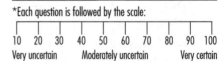

| 10 | 20 | 30 | 40 | 50 | 60 | 70 | 80 | 90 | 100 |
Very uncertain   Moderately uncertain   Very certain

Each subscale is scored separately, by taking the mean of the subscale items. If one-fourth or less of the data is missing, the score is a mean of the completed data. If more than one-fourth of the data is missing, no score is calculated. (The authors invite others to use the scale and would appreciate being informed of study results.)

Source: Lorig, K., et al. (1989). Development and evaluation of a scale to measure perceived self-efficacy in patients with arthritis. *Arthritis & Rheumatism 32,* 37–44. Reprinted by permission of John Wiley & Sons, Inc.

FIGURE 3.1

The Rheumatoid Arthritis Self-Efficacy (RASE) Questionnaire

We are interested in finding out what things you believe you could do to help you with your arthritis. We want to know what you think you could do, even if you are not actually doing it at the moment. Please tick one column for each question.

Do you believe you could do these things to help you with your arthritis?

1. I believe I could use relaxation techniques to help with pain.
2. I believe I could think about something else to help with pain.
3. I believe I could use my joints carefully (joint protection) to help with pain.
4. I believe I could think positively to help with pain.
5. I believe I could avoid doing things that cause pain.
6. I believe I could wind down and relax before going to bed, to improve my sleep.
7. I believe I could have a hot drink before bed, to improve my sleep.
8. I believe I could use relaxation before bed, to improve my sleep.
9. I believe I could pace myself and take my arthritis into account to help deal with tiredness.
10. I believe I could accept fatigue as part of my arthritis.
11. I believe I could use gadgets to help with mobility, household tasks, or personal care.
12. I believe I could ask for help to deal with the difficulties of doing everyday tasks.
13. I believe I could do exercises to deal with the difficulties of doing everyday tasks.
14. I believe I could plan or prioritize my day to deal with difficulties of doing everyday tasks.
15. I believe I could educate my family and friends about my arthritis to help with the strains that arthritis can make on relationships.
16. I believe I could explain to friends and family when I do or do not need help.
17. I believe I could discuss any problems with my partner or family.
18. I believe I could make time for leisure activities, hobbies, or socializing.
19. I believe I could save energy for leisure activities, hobbies, or socializing.
20. I believe I could focus on the positive when I am feeling down.
21. I believe I could use relaxation to deal with worries.
22. I believe I could allocate time for relaxation.
23. I believe I could use a relaxation tape or instructions to help me relax.
24. I believe I could use regular exercise.
25. I believe I could be aware of my limits in exercise.
26. I believe I could manage my medication, knowing how and when to take it.
27. I believe I could look out for and avoid side effects of my medication.
28. I believe I could seek help with persistent side effects.

Likert scoring, strongly disagree to strongly agree, 1–5.

Source: Hewlett, S., Cockshott, Z., Kirwan, J., Barrett, J., Stamp, J., Haslock, I. (2001). Development and validation of a self-efficacy scale for use in British patients with rheumatoid arthritis (RASE). *Rheumatology 40*, 1221–1230. Used with permission from Oxford University Press.

FIGURE 3.2

with rheumatoid arthritis because the unpredictable fluctuations of its symptoms may contribute to feelings of helplessness. The Arthritis Self-Efficacy Scale (ASES) was developed to measure patient-perceived SE to cope with the consequences of chronic arthritis (Figure 3.1). Patients rate the strength of their perceived ability to perform each item on a scale ranging from 10 to 100 in steps of 10. Item scores are then summed, with a higher score indicating greater SE. A full description of the considerable evidence to support its psychometric properties may be found in Redman (2003).

A new measurement instrument (RASE) is available to measure SE in persons with rheumatoid arthritis specifically for those within the culture of the United Kingdom (Figure 3.2). Expert clinicians and patients developed items. Test-retest reliability was .7 at one week and .89 at four weeks. Constructed validity was tested against the ASES. RASE was sensitive to SM education programs (Hewlett et al., 2001). This beginning evidence of validity and reliability is encouraging.

References

Burckhardt, C. S. (1994). Arthritis and musculoskeletal patient education standards. *Arthritis Care & Research 7*, 1–4.

Edworthy, S. M. (2000). How important is patient self-management? *Bailliere's Clinical Rheumatology 14*, 705–724.

Hainsworth, J., Barlow, J. (2001). Volunteers' experiences of becoming arthritis self-management lay leaders: "It's almost as if I've stopped aging and started to get younger!" *Arthritis Care & Research 45*, 378–383.

Hewlett, S., et al. (2001). Development and validation of a self-efficacy scale for use in British patients with rheumatoid arthritis (RASE). *Rheumatology 40*, 1221–1230.

Keefe, F. J., et al. (2000). Understanding the adoption of arthritis self-management: Stages of change profiles among arthritis patients. *Pain 87*, 303–313.

Kruger, J. M. S., Helmick, C. G., Callahan, L. F., Haddix, A. C. (1998). Cost-effectiveness of the Arthritis Self-Help Course. *Archives of Internal Medicine 158*, 1245–1249.

Lindroth, Y., et al. (1997). A problem-based education program for patients with rheumatoid arthritis: Evaluation after three and twelve months. *Arthritis Care & Research 10*, 325–332.

Lorig, K., et al. (1998). Arthritis self-management program variations: Three studies. *Arthritis Care & Research 11*, 448–454.

Mazzuca, S. A., et al. (1997). Effects of self-care education on the health status of inner-city patients with osteoarthritis of the knee. *Arthritis & Rheumatism 40*, 1466–1474.

Mazzuca, S. A., Brandt, K. D., Katz, B. P., Hanna, M. P., Melfi, C. A. (1999). Reduced utilization and cost of primary care clinic visits resulting from self-care education for the patients with osteoarthritis of the knee. *Arthritis & Rheumatism 42*, 1267–1273.

Newman, S., Mulligan, K., Steed, L. (2001). What is meant by self-management and how can its efficacy be established? *Rheumatology 40*, 1–6.

Pimm, T. J. (1997). Self-regulation and psycho-educational interventions for rheumatic disease. In Petrie, K. J., Weinman, J. A. (eds). *Perceptions of health and illness*. Amsterdam: Harwood Academic Publishers.

Redman, B. K. (2003). *Measurement tools in patient education*, 2nd ed. New York: Springer Publishing.

Riemsma, R. P., Kirwan, J. R., Taal, E., Rasker, J. J. (2002). Patient education for adults with rheumatoid arthritis. www.cochranelibrary.com. Accessed 7/19/02.

Scholten, C., et al. (1999). Persistent functional and social benefit five years after a multidisciplinary arthritis training program. *Archives of Physical Medicine and Rehabilitation 80*, 1282–1287.

Solomon, D. H., et al. (2002). Does self-management education benefit all populations with arthritis? A randomized controlled trial in a primary care physician network. *Journal of Rheumatology 29*, 362–368.

4

Mental Health Self-Management

O f the 5 million Americans with serious and persistent mental illness, 40% to 60% reside with or receive care from their families. The current mental health system has failed to adequately address the service needs of these individuals and families (Doornbos, 2001). Although the term "self-management" is rarely used in the mental health literature, these patients and their families do indeed self-manage. Other terms sometimes used to depict elements of SM in this field include "coping" and "self-help." "Psychoeducation" is an internationally acknowledged term used to refer to interventions that combine imparting of information with therapeutic elements, social skills, relaxation; this term does not really conform to SM.

The full range of theoretical models for SM intervention cannot be found in the mental health literature, and measurement instruments for this type of disease are focused only on SE and not on lay beliefs, stages of change, or any of the other models introduced in Chapter 1. In addition, studies usually focus on one diagnostic class. There has, however, been progression toward a fuller model of educational services since the early days of psychiatric patient education programs, which were confined to education about medication management in an attempt to improve patients' adherence to medication regimens (Ascher-Svanum, Rochford, Cisco, Claveaux, 2001).

Standards for Self-Management Preparation
None could be located.

Effective Interventions and Measurement Instruments
SM preparation in mental health is available in written and computer format. Most is oriented toward diagnoses of depression and schizophrenia.

Depression Self-Management Preparation

Both bipolar illness and depression tend to follow a chronic course; many patients with mood disorders experience multiple episodes during their lifetimes (Cutler, 2001). Although most treatment for depression is delivered through primary care providers and facilities, many depressed individuals do not receive any health interventions. Exploration of the effectiveness of SM approaches for particular kinds of problems and individuals, frequently under the guidance of a health professional but much less expensive, offers the opportunity to make help more widely available.

Dowrick and others (2000) have studied the effectiveness of problem-solving treatment for depression, in which patients' symptoms are linked with their problems, problems are defined and clarified, and an attempt is made to solve them in a structured way. This simple, reproducible intervention can be delivered in the community without a complex health care infrastructure. Problem solving may be more acceptable to clients than are other treatments and, in this controlled trial, was found to be equally as effective as a course in prevention. The proportion of problem-solving participants who remained depressed at six months was 17% less than for the control group. This intervention reduced the severity and duration of depressive disorders and improved subjective mental and social functioning.

Another RCT found that the combination of problem-solving treatment and antidepressant medication was no more effective than either alone and could be delivered by suitably trained practice nurses or general practitioners. The problem-solving intervention was used to address and resolve patients' psychosocial problems, with the goal of relieving depressive symptoms (Mynors-Wallis, Gath, Day, Baker, 2000).

Although anxiety and depression are prevalent in primary care, not all practitioners possess the skills to do mental health work. A SM approach based on proven psychological therapies may widen access to effective treatment. Bower, Richards, and Lovell (2001) have reviewed trials of self-help intervention for patients with anxiety and depression in primary care. Table 4.1 describes the kinds of interventions tested. Although more rigorous trials are required, current reviews and meta-analyses of self-help treatments have suggested that they are more effective than is usual care in the short term. No economic analyses were available.

To date, studies have largely relied on written material; future evaluations should examine use of telephone and computer

TABLE 4.1 Interventions in the Review

Study	Study Groups	Description of Intervention in Each Group
Kupshik	Written material plus telephone contact with nurse	Information about anxiety, instruction in relaxation, managing worrying thoughts, and lifestyle changes. Contact with the project worker was to enable skill acquisition rather than to counsel. Contact occurred over a six-week treatment period. Project worker was a nurse supervised by a clinical psychologist.
	Written material plus biweekly meetings with nurse	As above, but with biweekly meetings in person with the nurse.
	Written material plus weekly meetings with nurse	As above, but with weekly meetings in person with the nurse.

(continued)

◈ TABLE 4.1   (continued)

Study	Study Groups	Description of Intervention in Each Group
Chalder	Self-help booklet and nurse advice	Three-part booklet with information about fatigue, self-monitoring and diary-keeping, and cognitive-behavioral techniques for overcoming fatigue, plus 10- to 15-minute discussion with nurse on the booklet and the patient's clinical assessment.
	Routine primary care	No further details.
Holdsworth	Self-help booklet	Booklet includes a range of techniques for anxiety, depression, and related complaints within the three systems model (of thought, feeling, and behavior); 42 pages, 7500 words, reading age: eight years.
	Routine primary care	Routine primary care with access to the booklet at trial end (although not clear that patients knew they would have access).
White	Self-help booklet	79-page booklet and double-sided relaxation tape ("deep" and "rapid") divided into information and treatment sections. Flesch score of 73 (fairly easy), estimated required IQ = 87. Meeting with psychologist involved assessment and 30-minute discussion of "Stresspac" and how to use it.
	Advice only	Same assessment as Stresspac group, but 30-minute description of self-help replaced by specific verbal advice on ways of coping while on the waiting list — e.g., importance of exposure, relaxation, and challenging negative thoughts. No written or taped material.

(continued)

◈ TABLE 4.1 (continued)

Study	Study Groups	Description of Intervention in Each Group
	No intervention	Assessment interview only, plus 30-minute discussion of the therapeutic intervention if appropriate.
		All subjects had a 90-minute assessment interview and were offered conventional cognitive behavioral therapy treatment at the end of the study.
Sorby	Self-help booklet and explanation by GP	Booklet describes anxiety in terms of causes of anxiety, intervention, coping strategies, and monitoring progress. GP registrar spent 10 minutes explaining contents.
	Routine primary care	Routine primary care, but no changes in medication in first two weeks and consultations at 2, 4, and 8 weeks after recruitment.
Donnan	Self-help booklet and cassette	Booklet (27 pages, 4000 words), Flesch score of 71, four sections (description of anxiety; stopping its development; coping with anxiety; summary), including patient quotes and diagrams. Audiotape (55 minutes) repeated material from booklet and contained expanded relaxation instructions.
	Routine primary care	No further details.
Milne	Self-help booklet	Advice about coping with anxiety, including causes and management (e.g., relaxation). Diagrams and self-test quizzes also included; 35 pages, with a Flesch score of 82 ("easy" level).

(continued)

◈ TABLE 4.1   (continued)

Study	Study Groups	Description of Intervention in Each Group
	Self-help leaflet	Summarized main points in booklet; 2 pages long, with a Flesch score of 69 ("standard level").
	Routine primary care	Routine primary care with promise of access to the most effective treatment at the end of the trial.
Kiely	Self-help leaflets	Six leaflets containing information on the causes, consequences, and control of stress, plus 3 minutes extra GP time to administer self-help package.
	Routine primary care	No further details.

Source: Bower, P., Richards, D., Lovell, K. (2001). The clinical and cost-effectiveness of self-help treatments for anxiety and depressive disorders in primary care: A systematic review. British Journal of General Practice 51, 838–845. Reprinted with permission.

resources, expecially for patients with limited literacy. Structured self-help materials in any of these forms are available at any time. They provide skills in improving unhelpful thinking, poor problem solving, lack of assertiveness skills, and inability to take antidepressants.

Generally, studies examining outcomes of patients treated by self-help compare it with face-to-face therapy and have observed no signficant differences between the two treatments. Both are significantly better than a variety of control situations. Those that added practitioner contact while patients worked through self-help materials did not appear to benefit from this addition (Williams, Whitfield, 2001).

Perraud's Depression Coping SE Scale (DCSES) (Perraud, 2000) measures confidence that one can perform tasks designed to provide some control over depressive symptoms (Figure 4.1). Such an instrument could be used as an outcome measure for

Depression Coping Self-Efficacy Scale

Instructions:

The following measure describes coping activities that may be helpful in treating the symptoms of depression. Using a pen or pencil, under the column headed CONFIDENCE, mark how confident you are that you could do each activity using a number from 0 to 100. These numbers mean that you are not at all confident or sure (0%) to completely confident or sure (100%) that you can do each of these things listed. You may use any number from 0 to 100%.

0	10	20	30	40	50	60	70	80	90	100
Not confident					Moderately confident					Confident

SELF-EFFICACY STEM	CONFIDENCE MARK 0–100%
I am THIS PERCENT confident that I will be able to do the following things that may relieve or prevent the symptoms of depression ⇒⇒⇒⇒⇒⇒⇒⇒⇒⇒⇒⇒⇒⇒⇒⇒⇒⇒⇒⇒⇒⇒⇒⇒⇒⇒⇒⇒⇒⇒⇒⇒⇒⇒	
1. Tell others how I feel in a socially acceptable manner.	
2. Be aware of my behavior and how it affects others.	
3. Refuse requests of others when I do not wish to do something that someone else wants me to do, including authority figures and strangers.	
4. Go to bed and get up at the same time every day.	
5. Plan pleasant things to do for my free time.	
6. Limit naps to 20–30 minutes during the day.	
7. Ask for help when I am having trouble understanding something because I am not concentrating well (like income tax and legal documents).	
8. Eat four servings of fruits and vegetables daily.	
9. Drink 6 to 8 glasses of water daily.	
10. Recognize when I am blaming myself for my symptoms and try to stop.	
11. Engage in some sort of creative activity such as writing, reading, drawing, playing music, or working on projects.	
12. Get together with at least one very close person when I am feeling lonely.	
13. Get up and do something relaxing if I cannot sleep, before trying again.	
14. Question whether it is reasonable to think this way each time I think about myself in a negative way or assume that I am no good.	
15. Take a bath or do some other soothing activity before bedtime.	
16. Take medication the way my doctor recommends.	
17. Exercise or do some active thing every day.	
18. Be aware of when I am thinking about myself in a negative way or assuming that I am no good.	
19. Laugh and try to find humor in my situation, in spite of my problems.	
20. Challenge the thought that suicide is the only way I can deal with my problems.	
21. Attempt to understand why I am anxious when I have anxiety.	
22. Keep a journal describing my mood or how I feel emotionally each day.	
23. Meditate or do relaxation exercises at least once a day.	
24. Become aware of those feelings that bother me so I can work on not letting them bother me.	

Source: Perraud, S. (2000). Development of the Depression Coping Self-Efficacy Scale (DCSES). *Archives of Psychiatric Nursing 14*, 276–284. Reprinted by permission of Elsevier.

FIGURE 4.1

SM preparation as well as an assessment tool to help target those areas in which assistance is needed to help the depressed person persist. Content validity was checked with experts. The instrument is written at a seventh-grade reading level. Internal consistency was rated at .93; test-retest reliability was .84 in a nondepressed population. Factor analysis showed one factor: DCSES scores were significantly negatively correlated with depression scores, supporting the instrument's validity.

Schizophrenia Self-Management Preparation

Schizophrenia affects 2.6 million people in the United States. It can no longer be viewed as a chronic, inexorably deteriorating disorder with little chance for rehabilitation or recovery. When individuals with even severe forms of the illness are evaluated 20 to 40 years after the disabling period of their illness, more than half are functioning in a reasonably normal way, but only if treatment and rehabilitation services are continuously provided to individuals and families. A shift from treatment to rehabilitation is under way (Kopelowicz, Corrigan, Schade, Liberman, 1998).

Unfortunately, many persons with schizophrenia — even those who benefit from medication — continue to experience disabling residual symptoms and impaired social functioning and will most likely suffer a relapse despite medication adherence. Hence it is necessary to integrate empirically validated psychosocial treatment into the standard of care for this population (Bustillo, Lauriello, Horan, Keith, 2001).

A mounting body of evidence indicates that individuals with schizophrenia have the ability to recognize personal symptoms associated with relapse and use various mechanisms in an attempt to manage their symptoms. Individuals who scored higher on measures of symptom recognition were more likely to employ SM methods and to use them more consistently than were those who scored lower on symptom recognition. Difficulty in concentrating, a preoccupied feeling, and a feeling of being watched were most frequently identified by participants (Kennedy, Schepp, O'Connor, 2000).

Today, more patients than in the past are treated in an outpatient setting and stay with their families. For this population, SM preparation for families is essential. A meta-analysis of the effect of family interventions showed a decrease in patient relapse and rehospitalization rates from 60% to 40% — significantly better results than with usual standard medical care — especially when the family interventions lasted more than three months. (Pitschel-Walz, Leucht, Bauml, Kissling, Engel, 2001). Some studies also show a decrease in family caregiving burden, better patient adjustment, and decreased costs for society with SM preparation. Psychoeducation has gradually become a basic treatment for all schizophrenia patients and their families and part of the usual care regimen, at least in the United States.

Results of studies on general patient education (overlapping with more focused SM preparation) for persons with schizophrenia are far from conclusive, however. Provision of information, discussion, role play, problem solving, communication training, training in medication management, social skills training, and training in relapse prevention are common education techniques. Outcomes of interest include relapse, symptom control, social functioning, and quality of life. The strongest evidence is for relapse and symptomatology, which under some circumstances can be influenced by SM (Merrinder, 2000).

A Cochrane summary of 10 studies of persons with schizophrenia or related serious mental illnesses found that any kind of psychoeducation intervention in subject areas that serve the goals of treatment and rehabilitation significantly decreased relapse or readmission rates at 9- to 18-month follow-up, as compared with standard care. No effect on insight was found (Pekkala, Merinder, 2002).

One common form of preparation is social skills training, which uses learning theory principles to improve social functioning by remediating problems in activities of daily living, employment, leisure, and relationships. Ideally, the improved skills will generalize to better community functioning and have a downstream effect on relapse and psychopathology. Social skills training involves breaking complex social repertoires into simpler steps, subjecting them to corrective learning, practicing through role playing, and applying them in natural settings.

Some versions focus on improving impairments in problem solving and information processing that are assumed to cause social skills deficits. Attaining interpersonal and coping skills can help individuals with schizophrenia become more resilient to stressors. Effective problem-solving skills also are correlated positively with social competence (Kopelowicz, Corrigan, Schade, Liberman, 1998).

Social skills training may include broader SM skills, including medication self-administration, negotiation with mental health providers, self-monitoring of ongoing psychiatric symptoms, independent completion of basic self-care behaviors, stress management, and self-control of anger and hostility. A wide range of preparation methods can be matched to the patient's level of functioning, from role playing with a trainer and practice in real-life situations, to a full behavioral protocol including shaping, prompting, and generalization to build and reinforce appropriate behaviors. Further resources may be found in Kopelowicz et al. (1998).

Evaluation can occur through naturalistic observation by constructing role-play tests in which skills must be demonstrated. Individuals who have substantial cognitive deficits and who show high levels of thought disorder and conceptual disorganization are poor candidates for most of the social skills training formats that have been developed to date.

Current evidence indicates that while social skills training improves social skills for up to a year, improved competence in the community does not result and no clear effects on relapse prevention or psychopathology are seen. Nevertheless, many RCTs assume optimal antipsychotic medical management, which may well not be the case (Bustillo, Lauriello, Horan, Keith, 2001).

Concentration problems may preclude some patients with mental illness from benefiting from self-study materials. The most outstanding cognitive dysfunctions in patients with schizophrenia are inattention, memory and executive functions such as problem solving, planning and integration of behavior, self-monitoring, and error checking (also affected by some treatment modalities). Some schizophrenia patients — perhaps as many as one-third — do not manifest any signficant deviance in cognitive functioning (Rund, Borg, 1999).

Self-Management Preparation for Other Disorders

There is some track record of using bibliotherapy, self-help audio cassettes, and computer-aided self-help system to treat obsessive-compulsive disorder (OCD), phobia/panic, and depressive disorders. In bibliotherapy, for example, the patient takes a standardized treatment home in book form and works through it more or less independently. Contacts with therapists are merely supportive or facilitative and occur through an initial meeting and follow-up phone calls. This approach seems most beneficial for patients who have mild to moderate depression but who are not suicidal (Cuijpers, 1997). Kenwright, Liness, and Marks (2001) describe a computer-guided self-help system (Fear Fighter) for phobia/panic sufferers that allows them to identify triggers for their panic and deal with it. Homework and problem solving is involved. Some of these approaches are very efficient in use of clinical time.

Marks and colleagues (1998) describe two studies of home-based self-assessment of OCD. Subjects were given a self-guiding manual and could use a touch-tone telephone to access computer-controlled interactive voice response interviews at their convenience from home. Using this system, patients rated themselves on OCD and worked out a plan for individually tailored self-exposure therapy. These studies included an initial diagnostic interview with a clinician and telephone contact with a coordinator.

An important element of SM for all persons with mental illness is learning to manage stigma. This occurs in a variety of ways, including conceptual framing of their illness as a biochemical or genetic phenomenon. For women with depression (Schreiber, Hartrick, 2002), adoption of this way of thinking (biomedical model) provided relief from a sense of shame and deviance and responsibility for becoming ill. This mode of SM, of course, limits the management of psychosocial factors important to their illness.

References

Ascher-Svanum, H., Rochford, S., Cisco, D., Claveaux, A. (2001). Patient education about schizophrenia: Initial expectations and later satisfaction. *Issues in Mental Health Nursing 22*, 325–333.

Bower, P., Richards, D., Lovell, K. (2001). The clinical and cost-effectiveness of self-help treatments for anxiety and depressive disorders in primary care: A systematic review. *British Journal of General Practice* 51, 838–845.

Bustillo, J. R., Lauriello, J., Horan, W. P., Keith, S. J. (2001). The psychosocial treatment of schizophrenia: An update. *American Journal of Psychiatry 158*, 163–175.

Cuijpers, P. (1997). Bibliotherapy in unipolar depression: A meta-analysis. *Journal of Behavioral Therapy and Experimental Psychiatry 28*, 139–147.

Cutler, C. G. (2001). Self-care agency and symptom management in patients treated for mood disorder. *Archives of Psychiatric Nursing 15*, 24–31.

Doornbos, M. M. (2001). The 24-7-52 job: Family caregiving for young adults with serious and persistent mental illness. *Journal of Family Nursing 7*, 328–344.

Dowrick, C., et al. (2000). Problem solving treatment and group psychoeducation for depression: Multicentre randomized controlled trial. *British Medical Journal 321*, 1450–1454.

Kennedy, M. G., Schepp, K. G., O'Connor, F. W. (2000). Symptom self-management and relapse in schizophrenia. *Archives of Psychiatric Nursing 14*, 266–275.

Kenwright, M., Liness, S., Marks, I. (2001). Reducing demands on clinicians by offering computer-aided self-help for phobia/panic. *British Journal of Psychiatry 179*, 436–439.

Kopelowicz, A., Corrigan, P. W., Schade, M., Liberman, R. P. (1998). Social skills training. In Mueser, K. T., Tarrier, N. (eds). *Handbook of social functioning in schizophrenia*. Boston: Allyn & Bacon.

Marks, I. M., et al. (1998). Home self-assessment of obsessive-compulsive disorder. *British Journal of Psychiatry 172*, 406–412.

Merrinder, L. B. (2000). Patient education in schizophrenia: A review. *Acta Psychiatrica Scandinavia 102*, 98–106.

Mynors-Wallis, L. M., Gath, D. H., Day, A., Baker, F. (2000). Randomised controlled trial of problem solving treatment, antidepressant medication, and combined treatment for major depression in primary care. *British Medical Journal 320*, 26–30.

Pekkala, E., Merinder, L. (2002). Psychoeducation for schizophrenia. www.cochranelibrary.com. Accessed 1/4/02.

Perraud, S. (2000). Development of the Depression Coping Self-Efficacy Scale (DCSES). *Archives of Psychiatric Nursing 14,* 276–284.

Pitschel-Walz, G., Leucht, S., Bauml, J., Kissling, W., Engel, R. R. (2001). The effect of family interventions on relapse and rehospitalization in schizophrenia — a meta-analysis. *Schizophrenia Bulletin 27,* 73–92.

Rund, B. R., Borg, N. E. (1999). Cognitive deficits and cognitive training in schizophrenic patients: A review. *Acta Psychiatrica Scandinavica 100,* 85–95.

Schreiber, R., Hartrick, G. (2002). Keeping it together: How women use the biomedical explanatory model to manage the stigma of depression. *Issues in Mental Health Nursing 23,* 91–105.

Williams, C., Whitfield, B. (2001). Written and computer-based self-help treatments for depression. *British Medical Bulletin 57,* 133–144.

5

Pain Self-Management Preparation

Pain is the principal reason patients see physicians. For nearly two-thirds of these patients, the pain is idiopathic in nature. Many of these pain sufferers are partially or totally disabled, sometimes permanently, and their poorly managed chronic pain frequently generates feelings of deep distress, hopelessness, and despair. Their condition is routinely undertreated in part because pain does not conform to the "scientific approach" to health and disease: It is subjective, its causal bases are poorly understood, it is not necessarily a symptom of an underlying physical problem, it doesn't fit the expert knowledge model, and no "magic bullet" for its treatment exists. Although medicine does attempt to relieve symptoms, the goal of therapy is to diagnose, cure, or prevent underlying diseases that produce symptoms. Thus, according to medicine's conceptual model, relief of pain is a secondary objective (Resnik, Rehm, Minard, 2001).

The majority of patients seeking health care for pain experience recurrent episodes of pain for a year or more, so once they are seen in primary care, pain frequently becomes a chronic or recurrent problem. For example, in the case of back pain, fewer than 15%

of patients will have a clearly identifiable organic pathology that adequately explains the cause of the pain (Ahles et al., 2001).

Patients with many disease processes must self-manage pain. For example, persons with pain associated with cancer stay at home for a great part of their disease period and must be skilled at handling their own pain problems (DeWit et al., 2001). Patients often hesitate to use medication, wait too long before asking for pain relief, and have difficulty reporting and communicating about pain.

In addition, there is a lack of agreed-upon criteria for adequate pain treatment.

Standards for Self-Management Preparation
None could be located.

Effective Interventions and Measurement Instruments
In one primary care setting, these patients were first seen by a nurse educator who assessed their pain and the psychosocial issues that often precipitate seeking care. Patient preference for type of pain management strategy was established and pain SM strategies were reviewed. Patients received written or audio SM materials by mail, along with a letter summarizing the problems identified and referring them to specific pages in the SM educational information. Patients were provided with problem-solving help for the psychosocial issues, accomplished through a worksheet and telephone interview. Patients defined the problem, listed pros and cons of potential solutions, and recorded the solution chosen. In the RCT of this program, persons in the intervention group reported much greater relief from medicine and other treatments, feeling they had good control over their pain and being satisfied with treatment, than did persons given usual care (Ahles et al., 2001).

Other pain SM programs have been community-based and nurse-delivered. LeFort, Gray-Donald, Rowat, and Jeans (1998) describe a RCT studying such a chronic pain SM program delivered in groups. This program was modified from the arthritis self-management program (ASMP; see Chapter 3) and delivered in 12 hours over 6 weeks. The content described in Table 5.1 was validated by health professionals who work with such patients. The treatment group made significant short-term

◈ TABLE 5.1   Chronic Pain Self-Management Program Course Overview

Topic	Session					
	1	2	3	4	5	6
Self-help principles	√					
Myths about chronic pain	√					
What is chronic pain?	√					
Balancing rest/activity	√			√		
Exercise for health		√	√	√	√	√
Pain management strategies (physical/cognitive/behavioral)		√	√	√	√	√
Depression			√			
Nutrition				√		
Evaluating nontraditional treatments					√	
Communication skills					√	
Medications						√
Fatigue						√
Problem solving	√	√	√	√	√	√
Contracting/feedback	√	√	√	√	√	√

Note: Course adapted with permission from Lorig, K., *Arthritis Self-Help Course, Leader's Manual and Reference Materials,* Arthritis Foundation, Atlanta, GA, 1992.

Source: LeFort, S. M., Gray-Donald, K., Rowat, K. M., Jeans, M. E. (1998). Randomized controlled trial of a community-based psychoeducation program for the self-management of chronic pain. *Pain 74,* 297–306.

improvement in pain dependency, vitality, aspects of role functioning, life satisfaction, SE, and resourcefulness as compared to the wait-list control group. Because the materials are based on a standard protocol, this kind of psychoeducational program can be reliably delivered in all communities and so made available to the at least one in ten adults who live with chronic pain, most often in the back, head, or joints. Over the past two decades, pain centers have been developed but access is usually by referral, is not available in all geographic areas, and remains costly.

Other programs have been developed for specific pain populations. Although low back pain accounts for significant numbers of health care provider visits every year, appropriate medical care and SM for this condition are still contested. Because educational interventions that teach only body mechanics and lifting techniques have not been consistently successful, new approaches are being tried. A model similar to the successful ASMP has been studied (Von Korff et al., 1998).

Four two-hour sessions led by group leaders who have back pain address specific worries about back pain (concerns about serious disease, long-term disability or chronic pain, major activity or movement that would exacerbate the problem), emphasize the safety and importance of resuming normal activities, and provide examples of patients who are effectively managing back pain in their daily lives. The intervention was not designed to decrease pain intensity but rather to mitigate worries and increase confidence in SM, which was accomplished in the experimental group. The authors suggest that engaging patients in problem solving about their back pain, enhancing SE, and addressing worries are the most potent elements in the intervention. Other similar interventions have also shown significantly decreased ratings on pain and interference with activities (Moore, Von Korff, Cherkin, Saunders, Lorig, 2000). Both of these programs were conducted in primary care settings.

This research found several common worries that should be addressed in every primary care back pain visit: the belief that a serious underlying medical condition might be causing the pain, concern that movement or activity could cause injury or increase pain, and concern that pain could result in long-term disability. The research also points to the potential for patients to assume greater responsibility for managing their back pain than is often expected by health professionals (Moore, Von Korff, Cherkin, Saunders, Lorig, 2000). Guidelines for non-specific low back pain advise minimizing medical intervention and resuming normal activities as far as the pain allows (Nordin, Welser, Campello, Pietrek, 2002).

Other interventions have specifically targeted cancer patients, an estimated 42% of whom suffer from poorly controlled pain. One intervention that proved successful in improving pain severity but not in decreasing functional impairment as a result of pain used a 20-minute individualized education and coaching session to increase knowledge of pain SM, redress personal misconceptions about pain treatment, set goals such as being able to sleep through the night and identify strategies to meet these goals, and rehearse an individually scripted patient–physician dialogue about pain control. The control group received standardized instruction in controlling pain. Patients had incorrect knowledge of how to take analgesics and they made the assumption that side effects could not be controlled and were worse than the pain (Oliver, Kravitz, Kaplan, Meyers, 2001).

Sample problems used in a problem-solving framework with persons with cancer pain are presented in Figure 5.1 (Loscalzo, Bucher, 1999). Self-appraised problem-solving competence has been found to be related to decreased pain, depression, and disability, suggesting that problem-solving training could be incorporated into pain management interventions (Kerns, Rosenberg, Otis, 2002).

Educational pain programs typically promote cognitive understanding of pain and pain models, and learning is frequently reinforced by self-monitoring procedures, diary-keeping exercises, and cognitive-behavioral strategies in which dysfunctional methods of thinking about and acting toward pain are modified.

An intervention with a different theoretical base (phenomenological epistemology and personal construct theory) focuses instead on possible relations between bodily symptoms, emotions and life situations, and change of focus from pain and disability to resources and potentials. Patients are urged to become

- The patient seeks to reduce pain by staying in bed and refusing to have visitors. Increased social isolation leads to increased depression and a sense of worthlessness.

- The patient and family want to save the drug for pain for times when the pain becomes worse. The irregular drug regimen leads to intermittent peaks of relief, valleys of pain, anxiety, and frustration.

- Family and friends reinforce the patient's worry concerning addiction to narcotics. Inadequate amounts of the pain-killing drug are taken, leading to pain, depression, and hostility.

- The patient's spouse is afraid to express dissatisfaction with the patient's pain relief to the prescribing physician. Withholding an open, honest assessment of the patient's pain leads to passivity, pain, frustration, and family conflict.

- Some respite care workers are reluctant to administer pain medications on a schedule "by the clock." Uneven doses cause sleeplessness, pain, fear of addiction, and hopelessness.

Source: Loscalzo, M. J., Bucher, J. A. (1999). The COPE model: Its clinical usefulness in solving pain-related problems. *Journal of Psychosocial Oncology* 16(3/4), 93–117. Reprinted by permission of The Haworth Press, Inc.

FIGURE 5.1   Sample problems related to pain that are amenable to a problem-solving intervention

aware of the experienced-based knowledge embedded in their bodies, so as to help them reconceptualize and reconstruct their ability to control pain, and to help them find skills that enable them to change the way they cope with pain, respond to bodily sensations, and deal with external demands. Experience-based exercises such as creative drawing, moving to music, guided imagery, relaxation, and awareness exercises are used to enable the participants to become more aware of how they construct themselves today and of possible ways of redefining and reinterpreting themselves.

In a RCT using this theory, after one year the intervention group reported significant decreases in pain, increased pain coping abilities, a higher reduction of health care consumption, and fewer persons receiving disability pensions than did the control group (Haugli, Steen, Laerum, Nygard, Finset, 2001). Other strategies taught to patients include attention diversion, relaxation procedures, cognitive restructuring, problem solving, goal setting and self-reinforcement, and use of nonpharmacologic pain management techniques such as cold, heat, relaxation, and massage. Significant others are taught principles of contingency management that encourage cueing and reinforcement of skills acquisition and practice and behavioral goal accomplishment (Kerns, Rosenberg, 2000).

In the past two decades, considerable evidence has accumulated that suggests the experience of chronic pain, emotional and behavioral correlates, and response to treatment can be signficantly influenced by beliefs and attitudes about the pain experience. Judgments of SE, perceived pain control, and catastrophisizing seem to constitute pain appraisals that are important in the adjustment to chronic pain. Maladaptive beliefs can become the internal reality controlling the patient's pain behavior and can be used to predict poor response to treatment; this suggests that belief modification represents an essential component of most successful treatment efforts. The belief that all pain is a "fire alarm"-type indicator of a specific physical pathology that, if only correctly diagnosed, can then be readily rectified via a medical procedure probably remains the core faulty premise lying at the heart of the chronic pain dilemma (DeGood, Kiernan, 1997–1998).

More than a dozen instruments have been developed to measure the cognitions, beliefs, and attributions that patients have about the course of their pain and their SE in dealing with it (deWit, vanDam, Litjens, Abu-Saad, 2001). Maladaptive beliefs have increasingly come to be recognized as a major risk factor in poor response to treatment for chronic pain, and change in beliefs has become more clearly linked to positive treatment outcomes. In the aggregate, pain belief instruments have been conceptually derived rather than empirically determined from a comprehensive sample of all possible pain beliefs. Most of the pain belief scales were developed and validated against concurrent measures with a minimum of attention being paid to treatment outcome or long-term follow-up. More work on these measures remains to be accomplished (DeGood, Kiernan, 1997–1998).

CHRONIC PAIN SELF-EFFICACY SCALE (CSES; FIGURE 5.2)

This instrument was fashioned from the Arthritis SE Scale, with similar factors: SE for pain management (alpha, .88); SE for

Chronic Pain Self-Efficacy Scale Items

Self-efficacy for pain management (PSE)

1. How certain are you that you can decrease your pain quite a bit?
2. How certain are you that you can continue most of your daily activities?
3. How certain are you that you can keep your pain from interfering with your sleep?
4. How certain are you that you can make a small-to-moderate reduction in your pain by using methods other than taking extra medications?
5. How certain are you that you can make a large reduction in your pain by using methods other than taking extra medications?

Self-efficacy for physical function (FSE)

1. How certain are you that you can walk one-half mile on flat ground?
2. How certain are you that you can lift a 10-pound box?
3. How certain are you that you can perform a daily home exercise program?
4. How certain are you that you can perform your household chores?
5. How certain are you that you can shop for groceries or clothes?
6. How certain are you that you can engage in social activities?
7. How certain are you that you can engage in hobbies or recreational activities?
8. How certain are you that you can engage in family activities?
9. How certain are you that you can perform the work duties you had prior to the onset of chronic pain?
   (For homemakers, please consider your household activities as your work duties.)

Self-efficacy for coping with symptoms (CSE)

1. How certain are you that you can control your fatigue?
2. How certain are you that you can regulate your activity so as to be active without aggravating your physical symptoms (e.g., fatigue, pain)?
3. How certain are you that you can do something to help yourself feel better if you are feeling blue?
4. As compared to other people with chronic medical problems like yours, how certain are you that you can manage your pain during your daily activities?
5. How certain are you that you can manage your physical symptoms so that you can do the things you enjoy doing?
6. How certain are you that you can deal with the frustration of chronic medical problems?
7. How certain are you that you can cope with mild to moderate pain?
8. How certain are you that you can cope with severe pain?

10 Very uncertain

.

.

.

100 Very certain

Source: Anderson, K. O., Dowds, B. N., Pelletz, R. E., Edwards, W. T., Peeters-Asdourian, C. (1995). Development and initial validation of a scale to measure self-efficacy beliefs in patients with chronic pain. *Pain 63*, 77–84.

FIGURE 5.2

coping with symptoms (alpha, .9); SE for physical function (alpha, .87); total score (alpha, .95). Participants indicate their perceived ability to carry out the specified activity or achieve specific outcomes related to pain management, coping, and physical function. Responses are recorded on a 10-point scale (by tens) ranging from very uncertain (10) to very certain (100). A scale score is the mean response for that scale (ranging from 10 to 100), and the total score (ranging from 30 to 300) is the sum of the scale scores.

Scores were significantly correlated with measures of depression, hopelessness, somatic preoccupation, and adaptation to the chronic pain. Patients with higher levels of SE reported less intense pain, less daily interference due to pain, greater perceived life control, less emotional distress, and higher activity levels than did patients with lower levels of SE. Research to date shows that SE beliefs are associated with chronic pain patients' level of functioning and response to treatment (Anderson, Dowds, Pelletz, Edwards, Peeters-Asdourian, 1995). Several of these findings were replicated in Arnstein, Caudill, Mandle, Norris and Beasley (1999): Higher pain intensity was associated with lower SE, and SE was negatively related to disability and depression.

Pain intensity and SE beliefs are consistently important predictors of disability in patients with chronic pain. This relationship is congruent with the notion that lack of belief in one's own ability to manage pain, function, and cope contributes to the extent to which individuals with chronic pain become disabled. CSES can be used to identify patients with low SE, so that a care plan can be designed to treat them; patients may need a structured approach to help them challenge their beliefs regarding how much activity restriction is appropriate given their actual physical limitations and their true risk for harming themselves through certain activities.

SURVEY OF PAIN ATTITUDES (SOPA; FIGURE 5.3)

Seven pain-related beliefs were assessed using the SOPA (Jensen, Turner, Romano, Lawler, 1994):

1. Belief in one's personal control over pain
2. Belief in the appropriateness of solicitous responses from one's family when in pain

Survey of Pain Attitudes (SOPA) and Scoring Key

Instructions: Please indicate how much you agree with each of the following statements about your pain problem by using the following scale.

0 = This is very untrue for me.
1 = This is somewhat untrue for me.
2 = This is neither true nor untrue for me (or it does not apply to me).
3 = This is somewhat true for me.
4 = This is very true for me.

1. There are many times when I can influence the amount of pain I feel.   0 1 2 3 4
2. The pain I usually experience is a signal that damage is being done.   0 1 2 3 4
3. I do not consider my pain to be a disability.   0 1 2 3 4
4. Nothing but my pain really bothers me.   0 1 2 3 4
5. Pain is a signal that I have not been exercising enough.   0 1 2 3 4
6. My family does not understand how much pain I am in.   0 1 2 3 4
7. I count more on my doctors to decrease my pain than I do on myself.   0 1 2 3 4
8. I will probably always have to take pain medications.   0 1 2 3 4
9. When I hurt, I want my family to treat me better.   0 1 2 3 4
10. If my pain continues at its present level, I will be unable to work.   0 1 2 3 4
11. The amount of pain I feel is completely out of my control.   0 1 2 3 4
12. I do not expect a medical cure for my pain.   0 1 2 3 4
13. Pain does not necessarily mean that my body is being harmed.   0 1 2 3 4
14. I have had the most relief from pain with the use of medications.   0 1 2 3 4
15. Anxiety increases the pain I feel.   0 1 2 3 4
16. There is little that I or anyone can do to ease the pain I feel.   0 1 2 3 4
17. When I am hurting, people should treat me with care and concern.   0 1 2 3 4
18. I pay doctors so they will cure me of my pain.   0 1 2 3 4
19. My pain problem does not need to interfere with my activity level.   0 1 2 3 4
20. My pain is not emotional; it is purely physical.   0 1 2 3 4
21. I have given up my search for the complete elimination of my pain through the work of the medical profession.   0 1 2 3 4
22. It is the responsibility of my loved ones to help me when I feel pain.   0 1 2 3 4
23. Stress in my life increases my pain.   0 1 2 3 4
24. Exercise and movement are good for my pain problem.   0 1 2 3 4
25. Just by concentrating or relaxing, I can "take the edge" off of my pain.   0 1 2 3 4
26. I will get a job to earn money regardless of how much pain I feel.   0 1 2 3 4
27. Medicine is one of the best treatments for chronic pain.   0 1 2 3 4
28. I am unable to control a significant amount of my pain.   0 1 2 3 4
29. A doctor's job is to find effective pain treatments.   0 1 2 3 4
30. My family needs to learn how to take better care of me when I am in pain.   0 1 2 3 4

FIGURE 5.3

31.	Depression increases the pain I feel.	0	1	2	3	4
32.	If I exercise, I could make my pain problem much worse.	0	1	2	3	4
33.	I believe that I can control how much pain I feel by changing my thoughts.	0	1	2	3	4
34.	Often I need more tender loving care than I am now getting when I am in pain.	0	1	2	3	4
35.	I consider myself to be disabled.	0	1	2	3	4
36.	I wish my doctor would stop prescribing pain medications for me.	0	1	2	3	4
37.	My pain is mostly emotional, and not so much a physical problem.	0	1	2	3	4
38.	Something is wrong with my body that prevents much movement or exercise.	0	1	2	3	4
39.	I have learned to control my pain.	0	1	2	3	4
40.	I trust that the medical profession can cure my pain.	0	1	2	3	4
41.	I know for sure I can learn to manage my pain.	0	1	2	3	4
42.	My pain does not stop me from leading a physically active life.	0	1	2	3	4
43.	My physical pain will never be cured.	0	1	2	3	4
44.	There is a strong connection between my emotions and my pain level.	0	1	2	3	4
45.	I can do nearly everything as well as I could before I had a pain problem.	0	1	2	3	4
46.	If I do not exercise regularly, my pain problem will continue to get worse.	0	1	2	3	4
47.	I am not in control of my pain.	0	1	2	3	4
48.	No matter how I feel emotionally, my pain stays the same.	0	1	2	3	4
49.	Pain will never stop me from doing what I really want to do.	0	1	2	3	4
50.	When I find the right doctor, he or she will know how to reduce my pain.	0	1	2	3	4
51.	If my doctor prescribed pain medications for me, I would throw them away.	0	1	2	3	4
52.	Whether or not a person is disabled by pain depends more on your attitude than the pain itself.	0	1	2	3	4
53.	I have noticed that if I can change my emotions, I can influence my pain.	0	1	2	3	4
54.	I will never take pain medications again.	0	1	2	3	4
55.	Exercise can decrease the amount of pain I experience.	0	1	2	3	4
56.	I'm convinced that there is no medical procedure that will help my pain.	0	1	2	3	4
57.	My pain would stop anyone from leading an active life.	0	1	2	3	4

SOPA Scoring Key:

Control: 1, 11*, 16*, 25, 28*, 33, 39, 41, 47*, 53

Disability: 3*, 10, 19*, 26*, 35, 42*, 45*, 49*, 52*, 57

Harm: 2, 5*, 13*, 24*, 32, 38, 46*, 55*

Emotion: 4*, 15, 20*, 23, 31, 37, 44, 48*

Medication: 8, 14, 27, 36*, 51*, 54*

Solicitude: 6, 9, 17, 22, 30, 34

Medical Cure: 7, 12*, 18, 21*, 29, 40, 43*, 50, 56*

* Reverse-scored items. Transform these items (i.e., 4 minus rating given) before summing with other items.

Source: Jensen, M. P., Turner, J. A., Romano, J. M., Lawler, B. K. (1994). Relationship of pain-specific beliefs to chronic pain adjustment. *Pain 57*, 301–309.

FIGURE 5.3 *(continued)*

3. Belief that medications, in general, are appropriate for chronic pain problems

4. Belief in oneself as unable to function because of pain

5. Belief in a relationship between emotions and pain

6. Belief that a medical cure exists for one's pain problem

7. Belief that pain signifies damage and that exercise and activity should therefore be restricted

Other authors have not been able to verify this factor structure (Tait, Chibnall, 1997).

Internal consistency for SOPA scales ranges from .7 to .84, and test-retest reliability from .8 to .91. A greater belief that hurt signifies harm, that one is disabled, and that solicitous responses from others are appropriate are associated with greater physical and psychosocial dysfunction and pain behaviors. Harm beliefs (the beliefs that hurt necessarily indicates damage and that activity should therefore be avoided) in particular were closely linked to measures of functioning and pain behavior. The belief that emotions affect pain is associated with psychosocial dysfunction (Jensen, Turner, Romano, Lawler, 1994). Harm belief scores are moderately to strongly related to all measures of patient functioning and behavior.

Some evidence indicates that the scale is sensitive to interventions (Jensen, Romano, Turner, Good, Wald, 1999). Two brief versions exist: SOPA-35 (alpha, .61–.81) (Jensen, Turner, Romano, 2000), and SOPA-30 (alpha, .53–.82) (Tait, Chibnall, 1997). The original SOPA is the most reliable version.

BARRIERS QUESTIONNAIRE (BQ; FIGURE 5.4)

Patients' reluctance to report pain and to use analgesics are considered major barriers to pain management. BQ assesses the extent to which they have concerns about reporting pain and using pain medication. Specific concerns include fear of addiction, beliefs that "good" patients do not complain about pain, and concern about side effects. Higher levels of concern were correlated with higher levels of pain, and undermedicated patients reported significantly higher levels of concern, which represents evidence of construct validity. Internal consistency

Barriers Questionnaire II (BQ-II)

We are interested in learning about your attitudes toward treatment of pain. We want to know what you think. Some of the questions may seem similar to other ones, but please answer all of the questions. For each of the items below, please circle the number (0, 1, 2, 3, 4, or 5) that comes closest to how much you agree with that item.

	Do not agree at all				Agree very much	
1. Cancer pain can be relieved.	0	1	2	3	4	5
2. There is a danger of becoming addicted to pain medicine.	0	1	2	3	4	5
3. Drowsiness from pain medicine is difficult to control.	0	1	2	3	4	5
4. Pain medicine weakens the immune system.	0	1	2	3	4	5
5. Confusion from pain medicine cannot be controlled.	0	1	2	3	4	5
6. When you use pain medicine your body becomes used to its effects and pretty soon it won't work anymore.	0	1	2	3	4	5
7. Using pain medicine blocks your ability to know if you have any new pain.	0	1	2	3	4	5
8. Pain medicine can effectively control cancer pain.	0	1	2	3	4	5
9. Many people with cancer get addicted to pain medicine.	0	1	2	3	4	5
10. Nausea from pain medicine cannot be relieved.	0	1	2	3	4	5
11. It is important to be strong by not talking about pain.	0	1	2	3	4	5
12. It is important for the doctor to focus on curing illness, and not waste time controlling pain.	0	1	2	3	4	5
13. Using pain medicine can harm your immune system.	0	1	2	3	4	5
14. Pain medicine makes you say or do embarrassing things.	0	1	2	3	4	5
15. If you take pain medicine when you have some pain, then it might not work as well if the pain becomes worse.	0	1	2	3	4	5
16. Pain medicine can keep you from knowing what's going on in your body.	0	1	2	3	4	5
17. Constipation from pain medicine cannot be relieved.	0	1	2	3	4	5
18. If doctors have to deal with pain they won't concentrate on curing the disease.	0	1	2	3	4	5
19. Pain medicine can hurt your immune system.	0	1	2	3	4	5
20. It is easier to put up with pain than with the side effects that come from pain medicine.	0	1	2	3	4	5
21. If you use pain medicine now, it won't work as well if you need it later.	0	1	2	3	4	5
22. Pain medicine can mask changes in your health.	0	1	2	3	4	5
23. Pain medicine is very addictive.	0	1	2	3	4	5
24. Medicine can relieve cancer pain.	0	1	2	3	4	5
25. Doctors might find it annoying to be told about pain.	0	1	2	3	4	5
26. Reports of pain could distract a doctor from curing the cancer.	0	1	2	3	4	5
27. If I talk about pain, people will think I'm a complainer.	0	1	2	3	4	5

FIGURE 5.4

Scoring the Barriers Questionnaire II

1. Items 1, 8 and 24 (Fatalism) are reverse scored before analysis.
2. The mean scores on the total scale (27 items) and subscales is used for analysis.

Subscale	Items	#
Physiological Effects		
	Drowsiness from pain medicine is difficult to control.	3
	Confusion from pain medicine cannot be controlled.	5
	When you use pain medicine your body becomes used to its effects and pretty soon it won't work anymore.	6
	Using pain medicine blocks your ability to know if you have any new pain.	7
	Nausea from pain medicine cannot be relieved.	10
	Pain medicine makes you say or do embarrassing things.	14
	If you take pain medicine when you have some pain, then it might not work as well if the pain becomes worse.	15
	Pain medicine can keep you from knowing what's going on in your body.	16
	Constipation from pain medicine cannot be relieved.	17
	It is easier to put up with pain than with the side effects that come from pain medicine.	20
	If you use pain medicine now, it won't work as well if you need it later.	21
	Pain medicine can mask changes in your health.	22
Fatalism		
	Cancer pain can be relieved.	1
	Pain medicine can effectively control cancer pain.	8
	Medicine can relieve cancer pain.	24
Communication		
	It is important to be strong by not talking about pain.	11
	It is important for the doctor to focus on curing illness, and not waste time controlling pain.	12
	If doctors have to deal with pain they won't concentrate on curing the disease.	18
	Doctors might find it annoying to be told about pain.	25
	Reports of pain could distract a doctor from curing the cancer.	26
	If I talk about pain, people will think I'm a complainer.	27
Harmful Effects		
	There is a danger of becoming addicted to pain medicine.	2
	Pain medicine weakens the immune system.	4
	Many people with cancer get addicted to pain medicine.	9
	Using pain medicine can harm your immune system.	13
	Pain medicine can hurt your immune system.	19
	Pain medicine is very addictive.	23

Source: Sandra Ward, PhD, RN; Sigridur Gunnarsdottir, MS, RN. Reprinted with permission.

FIGURE 5.4 *(continued)*

reliability ranged from .54 to .91 and was .89 for the entire scale; test-retest reliability ranged from .60 to .81 and was .9 for the entire scale (Ward and others, 1993). Total score is the mean of all items, scored from 0 (don't agree at all) to 5 (agree very much).

A version of BQ has also been developed for use in Puerto Rico, which shows internal consistency of .37–.8 (Ward, Hernandez, 1994), and another version for Taiwan, which shows internal consistency of .59–.91. These instruments were translated and back-translated. In both cases, patients who were not using adequate analgesic medication had higher BQ-PR and BQ-Taiwan total scores than those who did. After controlling for demographic and disease varibles, family caregiver barriers were found to be significant predictors of inadequate management of cancer pain (Lin, 2002).

A short version of BQ has also been tested; it shows internal consistencies of .7 (Ward, Carlson-Dakes, Hughes, Kwekkeboom, Donovan, 1998) or .67 (Ward, Donovan, Owen, Grosen, Serlin, 2000). A test of the sensitivity of BQ suggested that where individuals have well-established but medically unsound beliefs based on prior experiences, simple information provision may not be sufficient without first understanding patients' schemata of cancer pain.

PATIENT BELIEFS AND PERCEPTIONS INVENTORY (PBPI; FIGURES 5.5 AND 5.6)

Beliefs that represent a patient's own conceptualization of what pain means for him or her may be discordant with current scientific understanding, which is believed to affect the individual's ability to benefit from prescribed treatment. When pain becomes persistent, patients may abandon previously held cultural or personal beliefs to form new pain beliefs. Beliefs are best judged not by how true they are but rather by how adaptive they are in enabling the believer to function in the world he or she experiences.

PBPI assesses these new beliefs and can be used at critical points throughout the course of treatment. It consists of three

---

Pain Beliefs and Perceptions Inventory (PBAPI)

The following is a listing of the PBAPI items reorganized by their factored scales. Each item is associated with a 4-point Likert scale (e.g., -2 = strongly disagree, to 2 = strongly agree). There is no 0 point. Items that are starred are scored with inverted values so as to be consistent with the scale construct.

Pain stability (TIME)

*3. There are times when I am pain-free.

6. I am continuously in pain.

10. It seems like I wake up with pain and I go to sleep with pain.

16. My pain varies in intensity but is always with me.

2. I used to think my pain was curable but now I'm not so sure.

5. My pain is here to stay.

*9. My pain is a temporary problem in my life.

*12. There is a cure for my pain.

*15. Someday I'll be 100% pain free again.

Pain as a mystery (MYST)

1. No one's been able to tell me exactly why I'm in pain.

4. My pain is confusing to me.

8. I don't know enough about my pain.

14. I can't figure out why I'm in pain.

Self-blame (S-B)

7. If I am in pain it is my own fault.

11. I am the cause of my pain.

13. I blame myself if I am in pain.

Source: Williams, D. A., Thorn, B. E. (1989). An engineered assessment of pain beliefs. *Pain 36*, 351–358.

FIGURE 5.5

scales identified by factor analysis:

- Time: future-oriented beliefs that pain will be an enduring part of life (alpha, .8)
- Mystery: the idea that pain is a mysterious, aversive, poorly understood event (alpha, .8)
- Self-blame: the notion that patients are appropriate targets of blame for their own pain (alpha, .65)

Others have found four factors instead of three.

PBPI was originally developed with injured workers. Perception of constancy is associated with pain ratings. A higher permanence score is associated with decreased perceived coping effectiveness. Belief in mystery is associated with both anxiety and depression, and belief in self-blame for pain is

Pain Beliefs and Perceptions Inventory: Scoring Key

The PBPI can be scored in three ways.

1. Original (scale) scoring (Williams and Thorn, *Pain 36*, (1989) 351–358).

   Scales:

   TIME = 2 + 3(R) + 5 + 6 + 9(R) + 10 + 12(R) + 15(R) + 16

   MYSTERY = 1 + 4 + 8 + 14

   SELF-BLAME = 7 + 11 + 13

Note: R = Reverse scoring (i.e., $-2 = +2$)

Note: Positive scores indicate endorsement of the belief (e.g., the belief that pain will be enduring with time, the belief that pain is a mystery and the belief that blame for the pain should be directed toward oneself).

2. Cluster scoring (Williams and Keefe, *Pain 46* (1991) 185–190).

   Step 1: Score the PBPI using original scoring.

   Step 2: Equate (standardize) the scales by dividing the sum of each scale by the number of items in each scale.

   TIME = (sum)/9

   MYST = (sum)/4

   SB = (sum)3

   Step 3: Determine cluster.

   Cluster 1 (high TIME, low MYST)
   If TIME > 0 and MYST < 0, the subject falls into cluster 1.

   Cluster 2 (high TIME, high MYST)
   If TIME > 0 and MYST > 0, the subject falls into cluster 2.

   Cluster 3 (low TIME, low MYST)
   If TIME ≤ 0 and MYST ≤ 0, the subject is a member of cluster 3.

A few patients may not fit into any of the clusters described (e.g., low TIME and high MYST). This group is likely to be relatively small and currently behavioral corollaries do not exist to describe this theoretically possible yet empirically unvalidated cluster of patients.

3. Four-factor solution (IASP 7th World Congress on Pain, Topical Seminar, Paris, France, Aug. 1993).

   MYST = (1 + 4 + 8 + 14)/4

   PERM = (2 + 5 + 9(R) + 12(R) + 15(R))/5

   CONST = (3(R) + 6 + 10 + 16)/4

   SELF-BLAME = (7 + 11 + 13)/3

Source: Williams, D. A., Robinson, M. E., Geisser, M.E. (1994). Pain beliefs: Assessment and utility. *Pain 59,* 71–78.

FIGURE 5.6

associated with depression symptoms. PBPI is also available in German (Williams, Robinson, Geisser, 1994).

Suggested interventions for common belief clusters are described by Williams and Keefe (1991). Patients who believe that their pain will endure and is mysterious might be helped to believe that even if pain is not understandable, it can be influenced by effort. Those who see pain as enduring but have a good understanding of it tend to rate their ability to decrease pain by using coping strategies as low; they can be helped by significant improvements in mood, self-worth, and control. Those who believe that they understand their pain and that it will be of short duration respond best to cognitive behavioral interventions.

PAIN STAGES OF CHANGE QUESTIONNAIRE (PSOCQ; FIGURE 5.7)

A significant subset of individuals with chronic pain are not successfully engaged in treatment. This instrument is designed to assess an individual's readiness to adopt a SM approach to chronic pain. As would be predicted by the transtheoretical model, four factors were found, with those in the precontemplative stage scoring high in reliance on passive coping strategies and those in the action and maintenance stages showing significantly negative reliance on passive coping (Kerns, Rosenberg, Jamison, Caudill, Haythornthwaite, 1997). In two samples studied, 1% to 5% of pain patients were precontemplators, 59% to 67% were in contemplation, 8% to 23% in action, and 14% to 16% in maintenance.

As would be expected, treatment completers and SM non-completers differed across these scales, supporting the PSOCQ's validity. The action and maintenance scales were significantly associated with use of exercise and stretching, beliefs in ability to control pain, and the idea that one need not be disabled. Precontemplation scores were associated with belief that one has little ability to control pain, that one is disabled, that hurt equals harm, and that a medical cure will become available. Action and maintenance scores increased over the course of treatment, supporting sensitivity of the instrument, and changes

Item Composition of the Pain Stages of Change Questionnaire (PSOCQ)

Precontemplation
1. I have tried everything that people have recommended to manage my pain and nothing helps.
2. My pain is a medical problem and I should be dealing with physicians about it.
3. Everybody I speak with tells me that I have to learn to live with my pain, but I don't see why I should have to.
4. I still think despite what doctors tell me, there must be some surgical procedure or medication that would get rid of my pain.
5. The best thing I can do is find a doctor who can figure out how to get rid of my pain once and for all.
6. Why can't someone just do something to take away my pain?
7. All of this talk about how to cope better is a waste of my time.

Contemplation
1. I have been thinking that the way I cope with my pain could improve.
2. I have recently realized that there is no medical cure for my pain condition, so I want to learn some ways to cope with it.
3. Even if my pain doesn't go away, I am ready to start changing how I deal with it.
4. I realize now that it's time for me to come up with a better plan to cope with my pain problem.
5. I am beginning to wonder if I need to get some help to develop skills for dealing with my pain.
6. I have recently figured out that it's up to me to deal better with my pain.
7. I have recently come to the conclusion that it's time for me to change how I cope with my pain.
8. I am starting to wonder whether it's up to me to manage my pain rather than relying on physicians.
9. I have been thinking that doctors can help only so much in managing my pain and that the rest is up to me.
10. I have been wondering if there is something I could do to manage my pain better.

Action
1. I am developing new ways to cope with my pain.
2. I have started to come up with strategies to help myself control my pain.
3. I'm getting help learning some strategies for coping better with my pain.
4. I am learning to help myself control my pain without doctors.
5. I am testing out some coping skills to manage my pain better.
6. I am learning ways to control my pain other than with medications or surgery.

Maintenance
1. I have learned some good ways to keep my pain problem from interfering with my life.
2. When my pain flares up, I find myself automatically using coping strategies that have worked in the past, such as a relaxation exercise or mental distraction technique.
3. I am using some strategies that help me better deal with my pain problem on a day-to-day basis.
4. I use what I have learned to help keep my pain under control.
5. I am currently using some suggestions people have made about how to live with my pain problem.
6. I have incorporated strategies for dealing with my pain into my everyday life.
7. I have made a lot of progress in coping with my pain.

1 = Strongly disagree
.
.
.
5 = Strongly agree

Source: Kerns, R. D., Rosenberg, R., Jamison, R. N., Caudill, M. A., Haythornthwaite, J. (1997). Readiness to adopt a self-management approach to chronic pain: The Pain Stages of Change Questionnaire (PSOCQ). *Pain 72,* 227–234.

FIGURE 5.7

in PSOCQ scales were associated with improved outcomes (Kerns, Rosenberg, 2000; Jensen, Nielson, Romano, Hill, Turner, 2000). Measures of internal consistency ranged from .77 to .86; test-retest reliability over a one- to two-week period ranged from .74 to .88. Alphas for the scales were as follows: precontemplation, .70–.75; contemplation, .79–.87; action, .8–.83; and maintenance, .7–.77 (Jensen, Nielson, Romano, Hill, Turner, 2000).

The precontemplation scale characterizes a person with little perceived personal responsibility for pain control and no interest in implementing behavioral change. Contemplative scores will be a consideration of behavior changes alone with increased awareness of personal responsibility for controlling pain. The action scale measures the degree to which someone is actively involved in learning SM strategies to control pain. The maintenance scale assesses the extent to which SM techniques have been incorporated into daily life, combined with a strong sense of personal responsibility for pain control. PSOCQ may be used in ongoing assessment of individual stages of change and modifications in them, so as to establish stage-matched interventions and to refine treatment approaches (Kerns, Rosenberg, 2000).

Treatment emphasizes development of a SM approach to chronic pain through a process of reconceptualization of the problem as subject to personal control and mastery. In this way, it encourages an active, problem-solving perspective. Therapy generally proceeds through a series of phases starting from reconceptualization of pain as manageable and subject to self-control, followed by skills acquisition and skills practice, and finally promotion of behavior change and its maintenance.

Some individuals maintain strongly held beliefs that their pain problem is a medical one that requires medical attention and that pain SM is irrelevant, if not impossible (Kerns, Rosenberg, 2000). Some authors doubt that in its current form PSOCQ is useful clinically as a tool for classifying pain clinic patients into distinct stages; further work should establish its utility in this way (Jensen, Nielson, Romano, Hill, Turner, 2000). Others (Biller, Arnstein, Caudill, Federman, Guberman, 2000) found that precontemplation scores were the best single predictor, identifying 61% of the patients who completed a SM program and 65% of those who dropped out.

References

Ahles, T. A., et al. (2001). Panel-based pain management in primary care: A pilot study. *Journal of Pain and Symptom Management 22,* 584–590.

Anderson, K. O., Dowds, B. N., Pelletz, R. E., Edwards, W. T., Peeters-Asdourian, C. (1995). Development and initial validation of a scale to measure self-efficacy beliefs in patients with chronic pain. *Pain 63,* 77–84.

Arnstein, P., Caudill, M., Mandle, C. L., Norris, A., Beasley, R. (1999). Self efficacy as a mediator of the relationship between pain intensity, disability and depression in chronic pain patients. *Pain 80,* 483–491.

Biller, N., Arnstein, P., Caudill, M. A., Federman, C. W., Guberman, C. (2000). Predicting completion of a cognitive-behavioral pain management program by initial measures of a chronic pain patient's readiness for change. *Clinical Journal of Pain 16,* 352–359.

DeGood, D. E., Kiernan, B. D. (1997–1998). Pain related cognitions as predictors of pain treatment outcome. *Advances in Medical Psychotherapy 9,* 73–90.

DeWit, R., et al. (2001). Improving the quality of pain treatment by a tailored pain education programme for cancer patients in chronic pain. *European Journal of Pain 5,* 241–256.

Haugli, L., Steen, E., Laerum, E., Nygard, R., Finset, A. (2001). Learning to have less pain — is it possible? A one-year follow-up study of the effects of a personal construct group learning programme on patients with chronic musculoskeletal pain. *Patient Education & Counseling 45,* 111–118.

Jensen, M. P., Romano, J. M., Turner, J. A., Good, A. B., Wald, L. H. (1999). Patient beliefs predict patient functioning: Further support for a cognitive-behavioural model of chronic pain. *Pain 81,* 95–104.

Jensen, M. P., Turner, J. A., Romano, J. M. (2000). Pain belief assessment: A comparison of the short and long versions of the Survey of Pain Attitudes. *The Journal of Pain 1,* 138–150.

Jensen, M. P., Turner, J. A., Romano, J. M., Lawler, B. K. (1994). Relationship of pain-specific beliefs to chronic pain adjustment. *Pain 57,* 301–309.

Jensen, P. P., Nielson, W. R., Romano, J. M., Hill, M. L., Turner, J. A. (2000). Further evaluation of the pain stages of change questionnaire: Is the transtheoretical model of change useful for patients with chronic pain? *Pain 86,* 255–264.

Kerns, R. D., Rosenberg, R. (2000). Predicting responses to self-management treatments for chronic pain: Application of the pain stages of change model. *Pain 84,* 49–55.

Kerns, R. D., Rosenberg, R., Jamison, R. N., Caudill, M. A., Haythornthwaite, J. (1997). Readiness to adopt a self-management approach to chronic pain: The Pain Stages of Change Questionnaire (PSOCQ). *Pain 72,* 227–234.

Kerns, R. D., Rosenberg, R., Otis, J. D. (2002). Self-appraised problem solving and pain-relevant social support as predictors of the experience of chronic pain. *Annals of Behavioral Medicine 24,* 100–105.

LeFort, S. M., Gray-Donald, K., Rowat, K. M., Jeans, M. E. (1998). Randomized controlled trial of a community-based psychoeducation program for the self-management of chronic pain. *Pain 74,* 297–306.

Lin, C. (2002). Barriers to the analgesic management of cancer pain: A comparison of attitudes of Taiwanese patients and their family caregivers. *Pain 88,* 7–14.

Loscalzo, M. J., Bucher, J. A. (1999). The COPE model: Its clinical usefulness in solving pain-related problems. *Journal of Psychosocial Oncology 16*(3/4), 93–117.

Moore, J. E., Von Korff, M., Cherkin, D., Saunders, K., Lorig, K. (2000). A randomized trial of a cognitive-behavioral program for enhancing back pain self care in a primary care setting. *Pain 88,* 145–153.

Nordin, M., Welser, S., Campello, M. A., Pietrek, M. (2002). Self-care techniques for acute episodes of low back pain. *Best Practice & Research Clinical Rheumatology 16,* 89–104.

Oliver, J. W., Kravitz, R. L., Kaplan, S. H., Meyers, F. J. (2001). Individualized patient education and coaching to improve pain control among cancer outpatients. *Journal of Clinical Oncology 19,* 2206–2212.

Resnik, D. B., Rehm, M., Minard, R. B. (2001). The undertreatment of pain: Scientific, clinical, cultural and philosophical factors. *Medicine, Health Care and Philosophy 4,* 277–288.

Tait, R. C., Chibnall, J. R. (1997). Development of a brief version of the Survey of Pain Attitudes. *Pain 70,* 229–235.

Von Korff, M., et al. (1998). A randomized trial of a lay person-led self-management group intervention for back pain patients in primary care. *Spine 23,* 2608–2615.

Ward, S. E., et al. (1993). Patient-related barriers to management of cancer pain. *Pain 52,* 319–324.

Ward, S. E., Carlson-Dakes, K., Hughes, S. H., Kwekkeboom, K. L., Donovan, H. S. (1998). The impact on quality of life of patient-related barriers to pain management. *Research in Nursing and Health 21,* 405–413.

Ward, S., Donovan, H. S., Owen, B., Grosen, E., Serlin, R. (2000). An individualized intervention to overcome patient-related barriers to pain management in women with gynecologic cancers. *Research in Nursing and Health 23*, 393–405.

Ward, S., Hernandez, L. (1994). Patient-related barriers to management of cancer pain in Puerto Rico. *Pain 58*, 233–238.

Williams, D. A., Keefe, F. J. (1991). Pain beliefs and the use of cognitive-behavioral coping strategies. *Pain 46*, 185–190.

Williams, D. A., Robinson, M. E., Geisser, M. E. (1994). Pain beliefs: Assessment and utility. *Pain 59*, 71–78.

6

Cardiovascular Self-Management Preparation

  Self-management approaches are available for limited areas within the realm of cardiovascular disease management.

Hypertension Self-Management Preparation

Twenty-five percent of the world's adult population is hypertensive; among Americans 60 years and older, two-thirds have elevated blood pressure (Vidt, 2001). Although more than 43 million individuals in the United States have hypertension, fewer than one-third achieve adequate levels of blood pressure control (Boulware et al., 2001). Self-measurement of blood pressure (SMBP) is not yet widely practiced and very infrequently involves self-adjustment of treatment such as medications (Ashida, Sugiyama, Okuno, Ebihara, Fujii, 2000). Perhaps the major advantage offered by SMBP is that it takes into account the fact that blood pressure is extremely variable over time, being influenced by physical activity and mental stress. For this reason, frequent measurement is helpful. Measurement by a health professional often yields artificially high readings (the white coat effect).

A growing body of evidence indicates that tight blood pressure control improves the cardiovascular and microvascular complications of diabetes. While the current gold standard for 24-hour blood pressure is ambulatory monitoring, it is too expensive to offer for large groups such as those with type 2 diabetes mellitus (Masding, Jones, Bartley, Sandeman, 2001).

Because the association between blood pressure and cardiovascular risk is continuous, there is no threshold above which the risk suddenly increases. Until further trials document the predictive value of blood pressure level to target organ damage, 135/85 is considered the upper limit of normal. Office blood pressure measurement by a physician with a mercury sphygmomanometer remains the standard because its relationship with cardiovascular prognosis has been demonstrated. The optimal frequency of SMBP is not yet settled.

The measurement is done much as it is in a clinic and is detailed in Figure 6.1. After a five-minute period of rest, the patient is seated with the device cuff of proper size maintained at heart level using the upper arm with the highest blood pressure. Many automated sphygomanometers have memory devices to avoid misrepresentation of blood pressure values. They can be accurate within 2–4 mm Hg. Electronic machines will inflate, deflate, and record blood pressure automatically, which is especially helpful for persons with arthritis (Asmar, Zanchetti, 2000). They can also provide a printout of blood pressure measures with the time and date, or they may store data for later analysis (O'Brien, Beevers, Lip, 2001).

SMBP is used in routine follow-up of known hypertensive patients and in evaluation of blood-pressure-lowering medications in clinical trials. It has been found to be one-third less expensive than is management by office visit, and mortality from hypertension has been found to be more closely related to home blood pressure levels than to casual office blood pressure levels. Because the measurement is more accurate, the number of subjects required for clinical trials is decreased (Brook, 2000). In addition, use of SMBP is generally associated with better

User Procedure

- SBPM should be performed after a period of five minutes' rest.
- SBPM should be performed with validated fully automated devices.
- Use brachial artery occluding devices.
- Wrist monitors are unreliable.
- Device cuff must be at heart level on the arm with the highest blood pressure.
- Measurement frequency:

   Initial phase and the treatment period—one-week SBPM: two SBPM morning and evening.

   Long-term observation—minimum one week per quarter.
- Patient diaries are unreliable.
- Use printer or memory-equipped devices with possibility to store or transmit.
- Discard first-day readings.
- Use all other data to calculate the mean SBPM.
- Manual device may be needed when arrhythmias are present.
- SBPM should be performed under medical supervision.
- Patients should be trained in SBPM and reevaluated annually.
- SBPM suited for patients motivated toward their health management.
- Patients with physical or mental disabilities may be unsuited to SBPM.

Source: O'Brien, E., Beevers, G., Lip, G. Y. H. (2001). Blood pressure measurement, *British Medical Journal 322,* 1167–1170.

FIGURE 6.1

adherence to treatment. Eighty percent of those selected for SM can be taught to self-monitor (Asmar, Zanchetti, 2000).

Generally, data from the initial day of self-measurement are excluded. Measurements taken twice daily for several days in a two-week period are evaluated; drug response can be evaluated in this time or less instead of the usual four weeks. Subsequent treatment can be individualized by evaluating duration of drug action. Stable hypertensives monitor their blood pressure on the first day of the month and more frequently if readings are elevated (Denolle et al., 2000).

Standards for Self-Management Preparation

No standards for SM preparation could be located. In addition, no standard guidelines have been established regarding the proper interval for calibration of the measurement device.

Effective Interventions and Measurement Instruments

The 30-year-old National High Blood Pressure Education Program has been very successful in its goals of increasing diagnosis and control of hypertension (from 16% in 1972 to 64% currently). This program has no doubt contributed to the documented decreases in cardiovascular disease and stroke. It has not yet focused on SM or preparation for it, however (Jones, Hall, 2002). The group that it has not reached holds beliefs quite different from those of patients on SM or ambulatory/ clinic management. A study of African Americans on the street in Dallas found that 35% attributed high blood pressure to eating pork or other foods, believing that they make the blood travel too fast to the head. High blood pressure was seen as symptomatic and treatable with vitamins, garlic, or other herbs. Only 15% related hypertension to an elevated pressure in blood vessels (Wilson et al., 2002).

Reimbursement for equipment and provider interpretation of readings are essential components of any SMBP program.

Zarnke, Feagan, Mahon, and Feldman (1997) describe a RCT of home blood pressure monitoring involving subjects with chronic stable hypertension, in which patients adjusted their own drug therapy if readings consistently exceeded defined limits (see the algorithms in Figures 6.2 and 6.3). In comparison with office-based management through physician visits, the patient-directed management was significantly more effective in achieving the desired blood pressure change. On the other hand, a study of patients who had been self-measuring their blood pressure found inadequate knowledge and performance of the measurement technique, and inadequate equipment was commonplace. Studies of health professionals reveal similar problems. Efforts to standardize blood pressure measurement are necessary (Campbell, Milkovich, Burgess, McKay, 2001). Well-calibrated, memory-equipped, phone-linked sphygmomanometers can increase accuracy (Denolle et al., 2000).

NAME: **Ms. Y**   FAMILY DOCTOR: **Dr. B**

Antihypertensive Medications:

   Nifedipine GITS 90 mg once per day
   Atenolol 50 mg once per day

Is Your Blood Pressure Low?

1. If you need to decrease your antihypertensive medications, do so in the following order:

    1. Nifedipine GITS

    2. Atenolol

2. Is **BP** <110/and/70 for most of one week (at least 4 of 7 days)?
   DECREASE nifedipine GITS from 90 mg to 60 mg once per day.

3. Is **BP** still low? [<110/and/70 for most of one week (at least 4 of 7 days)]
   DECREASE nifedipine GITS from 60 mg to 30 mg once per day.

4. Is **BP** still low? [<110/and/70 for most of one week (at least 4 of 7 days)]
   DECREASE atenolol from 100 mg to 50 mg once per day.

5. Is **BP** still low? [<110/and/70 for most of one week (at least 4 of 7 days)]
   DECREASE atenolol from 50 mg to 25 mg once per day.

6. Is **BP** still low? [<110/and/70 for most of one week (at least 4 of 7 days)]
   CALL Dr. B at Telephone: 123-4567.

Source: Zarnke, K. B., Feagan, B. G., Mahon, J. L., Feldman, R. D. (1997). A randomized study comparing a patient-directed hypertension management strategy with usual office-based care. *American Journal of Hypertension 10,* 58–67.

FIGURE 6.2   A sample algorithm for possible downward adjustments of drug therapy, individualized to match the subject's medications at the time of enrollment

At present, SMBP is performed mostly by patients on their own initiative using devices bought without professional advice; instead, SM should be used by informed patients who remain under health professional supervision (O'Brien, Beevers, Lip, 2001). Although SMBP offers significant advantages, it must be accompanied by regular training and checks of accuracy. Self-treatment (particularly by means of medication adjustment) is not the norm. There is little information about

---

NAME: <u>Mr. X</u>   FAMILY DOCTOR: <u>Dr. A</u>

Antihypertensive Medications:

    Atenolol 50 mg once per day
    Hydrochlorothiazide 12.5 mg once per day

Is Your Blood Pressure Elevated? Yes?

1. If **BP** is greater than 160/or/95 for most of two weeks (at least 8 days of 2 wks):
    YES? INCREASE atenolol from 50 mg to 100 mg once/day.

2. After two weeks, is **BP** still elevated? (>160/or/95 for at least 8 days of 2 wks)
    YES? INCREASE hydrochlorothiazide from 12.5 mg to 25 mg once/day.

3. After two weeks, is **BP** still elevated? (>160/or/95 for at least 8 days of 2 wks)
    YES? See Dr. A. for consideration of adding nifedipine GITS 30 mg once/day.

4. After two weeks, is **BP** still elevated? (>160/or/95 for at least 8 days of 2 wks)
    YES? INCREASE nifedipine GITS from 30 mg to 60 mg once/day.

5. Is **BP** still elevated 2 weeks later? (>160/or/95 for at least 8 days of 2 wks)
    CALL Dr. A at Telephone: 123-4567.

Is Your Blood Pressure Elevated? No?

If Normal? Continue your medications unchanged.

If <110/and/70? See "Is your blood pressure low?"

Source: Zarnke, K. B., Feagan, B. G., Mahon, J. L., Feldman, R. D. (1997). A randomized study comparing a patient-directed hypertension management strategy with usual office-based care. *American Journal of Hypertension 10,* 58–67.

FIGURE 6.3   A sample algorithm for possible upward adjustments of drug therapy, individualized to match the subject's medications at the time of enrollment

preparation for SM, the characteristics of those who cannot learn to do so, and other instructional methods that might prove successful.

Stroke Self-Management Preparation

Approximately 600,000 people experience a new or recurrent stroke each year. Approximately 3 million Americans are living with various degrees of disability from stroke, making it the major reason for disability in the United States. Post-stroke effects include hemiparesis, poor balance, aphasia, bowel and bladder problems, visual difficulties, and speech and memory problems. Because stroke is an event that may involve significant impairment of basic functions, post-stroke management is seen as rehabilitation rather than as SM.

Evidence indicates that after discharge from an acute rehabilitation program, stroke survivors do not have access to adequate SM preparation and lose ground in many areas of self-care (Johnson, Pearson, 2000). Yet after rehabilitation, SM is crucial and for those patients with little impairment may constitute the only preparation they will receive. Educational programs offered during the acute rehabilitation phase are most often geared toward family members. Stroke survivors who have returned home face issues that have yet to be adequately addressed.

It is reasonable to expect that SM preparation would be a potentially useful investment. Twenty to twenty-seven percent of stroke survivors are rehospitalized within one year of their initial stroke (Ottenbacher et al., 2001), and self-care ability as measured by the Functional Independence Measure (FIM) is significantly predictive of which persons would be rehospitalized. Given that prospective payment systems have been introduced for rehabilitative care, prediction and avoidance of preventable readmissions become fiscally significant.

There also is interest in enhancing recovery beyond the expected neural recovery. Using modified subscales from the Strategies Used by Patients to Promote Health (SUPPH) measurement instrument, which was developed by Lev and Owen and described in Chapter 2, Robinson-Smith (2002) showed that patient quality of life and recovery for stroke survivors are enhanced when self-care SE is high and that about half of the variance in depression is predicted by self-care SE.

Standards for Self-Management Preparation

In a review of post-stroke rehabilitation guidelines, Boult and Brummel-Smith (1997) found limited evidence for efficacy of rehabilitation programs and individual interventions. More than half of the literature citations showed no significant improvements in outcomes, although the guidelines imply that some stroke survivors do not receive rehabilitation from which they might benefit. SM preparation is not addressed except to note that caregivers should receive thorough training in techniques and problem-solving approaches to provide effective support.

Effective Interventions and Measurement Instruments
None could be located.

Anticoagulation Self-Management Preparation

Oral anticoagulation is designed to minimize the risks of thromboembolism, but the treatment itself constitutes a delicate balance between two serious complications: thromboembolism due to undertreatment and bleeding due to overtreatment. Tight control of the intensity of anticoagulation is therefore mandatory. A number of studies have clearly demonstrated that the number of complications increases in tandem with the amount of time patients spend outside the therapeutic targeted range (Christensen, Attermann, Hjortdal, Maegaard, Hasenkam, 2001).

Patients on chronic anticoagulation therapy require regular monitoring of the prothrombin time (PT) and mandatory individual dose adjustment to ensure that PT remains within the therapeutic range (see Table 6.1). The biological effects of Warfarin or Coumarin derivatives are extremely variable, both inter- and intra-individually, because of fluctuating bioavailability, inconsistent dietary vitamin K intake, changes in other drugs the patient may be taking, and variable binding to plasma proteins (Cromheecke et al., 2000). Traditionally, this issue has been managed through outpatient clinics. Portable monitors that perform coagulation tests allow patients to test at home from whole blood obtained by finger stick, interpret the results, and self-adjust the anticoagulant dose.

Patients who self-manage consistently spend more time in the therapeutic target range than do those cared for in primary care or even in specialized anticoagulant clinics and have fewer

TABLE 6.1   Protocol Used by Patients to Adjust Dose of Warfarin[a]

INR Value Obtained	Action Taken by Patient
< 1.5	Contact doctor for advice
1.5–1.9	Increase dose of warfarin by 1 mg daily
2.0–2.5	Same dose of warfarin
2.6–4.0	Decrease dose of warfarin by 1 mg daily
>4.0	Contact doctor for advice

[a] If the patient fluctuated between ranges very often, the dose increment was changed to 0.5 mg daily rather than 1 mg.

INR = international normalized ratio.

Source: Sidhu, P., O'Kane, H. O. (2001). Self-managed anticoagulation: Results from a two-year prospective randomized trial with heart valve patients. *Annals of Thoracic Surgery 72,* 1523–1527.

thrombotic or hemorrhagic episodes. Patients should be in their own therapeutic range for at least 60% of the time (Fitzmaurice, Machin, 2001). SM is now a validated concept in selected adults (Christensen, Attermann, Hjortdal, Maegaard, Hasenkam, 2001).

Standards for Self-Management Preparation
None in English could be located. Standards are available in German (Taborski, Muller-Berghaus, 1999).

Effective Interventions and Measurement Instruments
Preparation for SM has been as brief as two two-hour sessions that included measurement in the presence of the instructor and practice in devising proper oral coagulation dosing. Content also included how drugs, diet, alcohol, and infection may alter coagulation. A 24-hour help desk was infrequently consulted. In general, all patients who are able to lead an independent and self-supporting life are believed to be capable of SM of

Protocol Used by Patients to Adjust Dose of Warfarin	
INR Value Obtained	Action Taken by Patient
<1.5	Contact doctor for advice
1.5–1.9	Increase dose of Warfarin by 1 mg daily
2.0–2.5	Same dose of Warfarin
2.6–4.0	Decrease dose of Warfarin by 1 mg daily
>4.0	Contact doctor for advice

Note: If the patient fluctuated between ranges very often, the dose increment was changed to 0.5 mg daily rather than 1 mg.

INR = international normalized ratio.

Source: Sidhu, P., O'Kane, H. O. (2001). Self-managed anticoagulation: Results from a two-year prospective randomized trial with heart valve patients. Annals of Thoracic Surgery 72, 1523–1527. Reprinted with permission from Society of Thoracic Surgeons.

FIGURE 6.4

anticoagulation, irrespective of their educational background and social status. Manual coordination and sufficient visual capability are needed as the patient has to prick his or her warm, clean, dry finger and place the blood drop exactly on the marked point of a test strip (Cromheecke et al., 2000).

Other SM preparation programs also focus on ways to recognize the side effects of over- and under-anticoagulation, hand hygiene while performing the tests to reduce risk of infection, and use of a protocol for patients to adjust Warfarin dosage (see Figure 6.4). Patients were encouraged to perform more frequent measurements if they had started a new medication, consumed more than usual amounts of alcohol, had unstable international normalized ratios (INRs), or had an infection (Sidu, O'Kane, 2001).

In Germany, 50,000 patients currently self-manage their own anticoagulation; they are prepared for this responsibility through nationally approved and formalized programs in 600 training centers. Nearly half require this treatment as the result of heart valve replacement. Fifty to sixty percent of all patients on anticoagulation were judged to be suitable candidates for SM (Taborski, Muller-Berghaus, 1999). Many

Association of Self-Management of Anticoagulation Training Course for Patients

Theoretical session

- Theoretical aspects of anticoagulation management
- Indications for anticoagulation
- How to monitor the blood
- Frequency of coagulation monitoring
- Problems with monitoring
- Interaction between anticoagulants and other drugs
- The influence of nutrition, alcohol, intercurrent illness, and travel on the efficacy of anticoagulants
- How to record the test results
- How to recognize and treat complications
- Overlapping heparin therapy
- Vaccinations
- Endocarditis prophylaxis

Practical session

- Operating the coagulation monitor
- Practicing a coagulation test
- Practicing an internal quality control test
- Correct finger stick procedure
- Possible sources of error
- Recording test results

Source: Fitzmaurice, D. A., Machin, S. J., on behalf of the British Society of Haematology Task Force for Haemostasis and Thrombosis (2001). Recommendations for patients undertaking self management of oral anticoagulation. *British Medical Journal 323,* 985–989.

FIGURE 6.5

patients needed as many as 20 attempts during several training sessions before they achieved success.

Content of one anticoagulation SM program may be found in Figure 6.5. At the end of the training, patients are "testified" to have met standards of the Association of Self-Management of Anticoagulation and obtain a certificate necessary for reimbursement for a monitor, test strips, and other items. Once competence has been established, it can take two to three months before patients are fully accustomed to managing their own treatment (Fitzmaurice, Machin, 2001; Morsdorf et al., 1999).

Little is known about the nature of patients' interpretations of their INR or their own quality control. The instrument must be checked for accuracy at least once a month and the patient's procedures and interpretation every six months (Fitzmaurice, Machin, 2001). SM is known to be more cost-effective than the alternatives.

As in many other areas, patient information on anticoagulation had a readability level of 10.7, with none of the materials at or below the sixth-grade level and 4% at higher than a twelfth-grade reading level. Note that 21% of the U.S. adult population has only rudimentary reading and writing skills, with elderly persons especially at risk for low literacy (Estrada, Hyrniewicz, Higgs, Collins, Byrd, 2000).

A RCT by Koertke, Minami, Bairaktaris, Wagner, and Koerfer (2000) provides an example of how SM preparation fits into the care process. Thromboembolism and anticoagulant-induced hemorrhage account for 75% of all complications following mechanical heart valve replacement. These complications occur most frequently during the six months following surgery; the risk then becomes low and remains constant for years. In this RCT, patients began training 6 to 11 days postoperatively. Eighty percent of the time these patients were in the therapeutic range, compared with 62% for the INR values monitored by family practitioners; their rates of severe hemorrhagic and thromboembolic complications were also significantly lower. Ninety-two percent of the study participants who began INR SM were capable of maintaining it over the long term. Only 8% of patients trained in SM were unable to continue it.

Other trials show that of 51 potential trainees, 6 didn't want to be trained, 3 were unsuitable because they could not get blood samples or manage dosing, and by the end of three months 6 had abandoned SM. After two years, 34 of the 51 remained in the program (Sidu, O'Kane, 2001). The performance of all who continued SM was regularly monitored even after the training period ended, however. Others (Fitzmaurice, Machin, 2001) suggest that SM patients must be reviewed by the responsible clinician at least every six months and external control procedures performed (the patient checks the INR on his or her own equipment and on the clinic's coagulometer). If the INR deviates by more than .5, the patient's technique and device must be reassessed.

Anticoagulation Self-Management Preparation in Children

While SM of oral anticoagulation has been validated in adults, it is unusual to attempt it with children. Christensen, Attermann, Hjortdal, Maegaard, and Hasenkam (2001) developed such a program for children requiring implantation of a mechanical heart valve because of congenital valvular disease. It appeared to be more difficult for children to stay within the targeted INR range (median of 66% of the time, but with a range of 17.6% to 90.4%) than is usual with adults (80% or higher). In children, the ratio shows greater fluctuation because their metabolic rate is higher and may be more susceptible to medication, food, and infection than is the case for adults.

During the entire study the equipment was regularly monitored every fourth week, and every six months the coagulometer was mailed to a hospital lab for a check-up. Both the children and the parents were satisfied with SM. Obviously some did much better than others (see range above)—the question then becomes how to select them.

In general, INR SM represents a highly significant improvement over conventional management (Koertke, Minami, Bairaktaris, Wagner, Koerfer, 2000).

Heart Failure Self-Management Preparation

Heart failure is the most common Medicare diagnosis-related group, and more Medicare dollars are spent on it than for any other diagnosis. One in ten elderly people suffer from heart failure, a clinical syndrome in which progressively deteriorating ventricular function results in vasoconstriction, fluid retention, marked activity intolerance from dyspnea and fatigue, impaired quality of life, and premature death (Moser, 2000). These patients typically move between health care sectors, being repeatedly admitted and discharged from each. In the U.S. health care system, in which institutional and community health sectors are separately organized, separately funded, and poorly linked at the point of service delivery, these patients are at high risk for discontinuity of care (Harrison et al., 2002).

Heart failure is frequently not managed optimally. Effective therapies are underprescribed. Exercise is rarely prescribed and dietary advice infrequently given. Most patients have little knowledge of their condition or its treatment. These patients are said to have a worse prognosis than those with most cancers and carry a heavy burden of illness (Blue et al., 2001).

SM of heart failure primarily focuses on optimizing drugs, diet, exercise, and early detection of decompensation. Apparently preparation for SM must be supplemented by regular health professional contacts, frequently by phone and for one year or longer, so as to detect clinical deterioration and to adjust treatment. The goal — to decrease expensive hospitalizations often due to fluid overload and to increase quality of life — has been well demonstrated (Cline, Israelsson, Willenheimer, Broms, Erhardt, 1998; Fonarow et al., 1997). Without this kind of care, more than half of all such patients are readmitted to the hospital within six months; half of these hospitalizations are believed to be preventable.

SM is difficult because early symptoms are subtle and treatment regimens are complex. In one group (Carlson, Riegel, Moser, 2001), only 45% of patients rated shortness of breath at rest as highly important. Those with sudden weight gain must decrease sodium and fluid intake and increase diuretic dose. In the elderly, the initial change may be decreased mental function noted primarily by the caregiver. Fewer than half of the group felt very or highly confident in their ability to relieve symptoms, and 59% felt little or no self-confidence in their ability to evaluate their actions. Patients were confused about seemingly contradictory advice to exercise and advice to rest.

Because of multiple comorbidities with related symptoms, patients need dietary, exercise, and other advice that is synthesized for all of their illnesses and yet specific enough that they will know exactly what to do. It is common for patients not to weigh themselves daily, not to know their recommended limit of daily sodium intake, and to forget to take or run out of their medication. Patients with little confidence in their abilities to sucessfully perform SM may delay seeking help until their symptoms clearly indicate that something serious is happening, at which point they simply go to the emergency department and require rehospitalization (Carlson, Riegel, Moser, 2001).

Standards for Self-Management Preparation
None could be located.

Effective Interventions and Measurement Instruments
The most common symptoms with heart failure are the following: shortness of breath; diuretic-related symptoms; swelling; decrease in concentration, attention, and memory; loss of balance and falling; chest pain; tiredness and trouble sleeping; and (more in women) fear, depression, and sadness. These symptoms were very problematic for patients (meaning they are not well controlled) and were self-managed largely by changes in physical activity, position, and temperature; medication management; adherence to a sodium-restricted diet; self-monitoring; and distraction techniques (Bennett, Cordes, Westmoreland, Castro, Donnelly, 2000). Content from a SM program may be found in Table 6.2 (Dunbar, Jacobson, Deaton, 1998).

Patients with heart failure frequently are cognitively impaired, making family preparation especially important. In a sample of community-dwelling patients with heart failure, cognitive impairment was present in 29% (Riegel et al., 2002b).

A summary of trials of disease management programs for heart failure, involving SM preparation and specialized follow-up of medical management, dietary consultation, and home visits, found a 13% lower risk of hospitalization for participants than for those receiving usual care. Unfortunately, there are 5 million heart failure patients in the United States but only approximately 150 such comprehensive programs (Ahmed, 2002).

A successful intervention (Fonarow et al., 1997) involved a flexible diuretic regimen, empowering the patient to correlate

TABLE 6.2   Comprehensive Congestive Heart Failure Patient Education

Teaching Content	Self-Monitoring Behaviors
Signs and symptoms to be reported to RN/MD	Calls RN/MD promptly at new onset or change in severity of symptoms: weight gain >2 lb within 1–2 days, shortness of breath, chest pain, edema, abdominal bloating, dizziness, nausea, fatigue, racing heartbeat
Daily weights	Purchases scale and weighs each morning after urination and before breakfast (in similar-weight clothing)
Sodium restriction (≤2 g per day)	Reads nutrition labels and limits sodium intake Finds acceptable sodium alternatives Sets dietary goals and rewards self for adherence Monitors sodium intake
Fluid restriction (≤2000 mL per day)	Measures and records daily fluid intake in milliliters Manages thirst
Medication regimen	Consistently follows prescribed medication schedule Adjusts supplement diuretic dose based on morning weight Monitors supply and plans for refills Has a system (pill box, routine time) for enhancing and monitoring own compliance
Caffeine restriction	Limits self to no more than two servings of caffeinated beverages per day
ETOH restriction	Avoids (if alcoholic history) or limits to 2 drinks/week Uses minimal alcohol and for special occasions only (weddings, etc.)
Smoking cessation	Sets smoking cessation goal and plan Works toward no use of cigarettes or tobacco

Desired Outcome	Possible Reasons for Noncompliance
Verbalizes understanding of how and when to call RN/MD	Denial, anxiety, fatigue, pain, unreceptiveness, cognitive/sensory impairment, and communication barriers
Identifies the cause of CHF symptoms such as fluid overload	
Weighs and records weight daily	Does not own scale
	Cannot read scale
	Cannot balance to stand on scale
	Cannot afford to purchase scale
Verbalizes understanding of diet restriction and demonstrates label reading	Inability to shop and prepare fresh foods
	Use of canned and frozen foods
Identifies the relationship between sodium intake and fluid retention	Eating "fast foods"
	Eating in restaurants frequently
	Literacy issues
	Cultural influences that support high-sodium foods
Demonstrates how to read labels and convert from milliliters to ounces and measures liquid intake	Feelings of thirst and the physiologic craving for increased fluid intake
Identifies fluid alternatives when thirsty	Doesn't count semisolid food (Jell-O, ice cream) as fluid
Follows prescribed medication regimen	Financial limitations
Verbalizes desired effects of drugs, usual side effects, and side effects to report	Real or perceived side effects
States relationship between daily weight and indications to alter daily diuretic dose	
Can identify beverages and foods that contain caffeine and the effects of caffeine on the heart	Caffeine addiction; possible attempt to battle the fatigue associated with CHF
Verbalizes understanding of how ETOH can decrease cardiac function	Alcohol addiction; possible attempt to avoid the feelings and issues associated with chronic illness
	Social environment
Identifies the dangers of smoking	Tobacco addiction

(continued)

◈ TABLE 6.2   (continued)

Teaching Content	Self-Monitoring Behaviors
Sleep and rest	Balances rest activity to manage fatigue
	Monitors symptoms of sleep disruption (orthopnea, nocturia)
Activity	Walks (as tolerated) or participates in supervised program
	Develops a consistent daily program of activity
	Avoids strenuous exercise, extreme temperatures, and heavy lifting

diet with fluid retention and making treatment decisions, thereby restoring some sense of mastery over a frustrating chronic illness. Patients were to respond to a two-pound or greater daily weight gain with an increase of diuretics and potassium. Education also addressed worsening heart failure, including arrhythmias and embolic events. Many patients had received specific instructions to avoid exercise, even though it is recommended in most heart failure programs and lack of it contributes to the deconditioning and sense of helplessness that often accompany advanced heart failure. Ongoing connection between the patient and the heart failure team is much more effective than is that triggered only by symptoms of deterioration.

A similar intervention (Harrison et al., 2002) focused on a nurse-led transition from hospital to home care and featured comprehensive patient education, proactive nurse follow-up, and increased access to providers including through home care. The structured protocol for education included a patient workbook and educational map. At 12 weeks post-discharge, 31% of the usual-care patients had been readmitted to hospital compared with 23% of patients in the special transition-to-home program; 46% of the usual-care group had visited an ED, compared with 29% of the transition group. Components of a suc-

Desired Outcome	Possible Reasons for Noncompliance
Identifies sleep hygiene strategies	Inadequate sleep hygiene
Understands the relationship between heart failure and sleep disruptions	Inactivity and/or excessive daytime napping
	Disruptive medication regimen
	Undiagnosed sleep apnea
Identifies the importance of regular exercise and states warning signals of when to stop or limit exercise routine	Physical disability/limitation or deconditioning

Source: Dunbar, S. B., Jacobson, L. H., Deaton, C. (1998). Heart failure: Strategies to enhance patient self-management. *AACN Clinical Issues 9,* 244–256.

cessful heart failure disease management program may be found in Figure 6.6. Case management via telephone has also been found to be effective (Riegel et al., 2002a); monitoring by way of home computers is being tested.

Other studies have also found significant success in using nurse home visits and telephone contact with the goal of educating patients for self-monitoring and management. Participants were given a pocket-sized book with full explanations; lists of their drugs, weights, and blood tests; and details of nurse contact and visits (Blue et al., 2001). Five other RCTs have found convincing evidence that in selected patient populations, decreased hospital admissions and days; increased quality of life, functional capacity, and patient satisfaction; and compliance with medications and diet could be attained, although most have occurred at academic centers and their generalizability to the broader population of heart failure patients remains unknown (Rich, 1999).

Virtually no research has considered SM preparation in the long-term care sector. To date, obtaining reimbursement for advance practice nurses to manage these patients has proved difficult.

Because this disease is difficult to manage and patients frequently are compromised in their learning ability, regular

---

Components of Successful Heart Failure Disease Management Programs

- Care managed by an experienced cardiovascular nurse with access to a cardiologist for consultation
- Vigilant, frequent follow-up after hospital discharge
- Increased access to health care professionals
- Optimization of medical therapy; patients prescribed appropriate drugs in appropriate doses using published guidelines based on large-scale randomized, controlled clinical trials
- Intensive, comprehensive patient and family/caregiver education about heart failure, emphasizing low-salt diet, medications, symptoms signaling worsening failure, weighing, and management strategies for problems
- Early attention to signs and symptoms of fluid overload (e.g., flexible diuretic regimen)
- Supplementation of in-hospital education with outpatient education
- Emphasis on addressing barriers to compliance

Source: Moser, D. K. (2000). Heart failure management: Optimal health care delivery programs. *Annual Review of Nursing Research 18,* 91–126. Used by permission of Springer Publishing Company, Inc., New York.

FIGURE 6.6

contact with many of these patients seems necessary to detect clinical deterioration, adjustment of treatment, avoidance of hospitalization.

SELF-MANAGEMENT OF HEART FAILURE QUESTIONNAIRE (SMHF; FIGURE 6.7)

This instrument was developed to be a clinically useful measure of the abilities of patients with heart failure to manage their disease. SM was defined as a cognitive decision-making process undertaken in response to signs and symptoms of heart failure and occurs in four stages:

1. Recognizing that a change in signs or symptoms is related to the illness
2. Evaluating the change
3. Implementing a selected treatment strategy
4. Evaluating the effectiveness of treatment

Self-Care of Heart Failure©

All answers are confidential.

SECTION A: How often do you do the following?

	Never or rarely	Sometimes	Frequently	Always
1. Weigh yourself daily?	1	2	3	4
2. Keep the salt in your diet lower than 2000–3000 mg (2–3 Gm) each day?	1	2	3	4
3. Exercise at least 3 times each week?	1	2	3	4
4. Take medications as prescribed?	1	2	3	4
5. Keep your weight within 10% of your ideal weight?	1	2	3	4
6. Talk to your doctor whenever you need guidance?	1	2	3	4
7. Get immunizations (such as a flu shot) every year?	1	2	3	4

SECTION B: Listed below are symptoms that people with heart failure may have. If you had a change in any of these symptoms, how *worrisome or troubling* would it be?

(circle **one** number for each symptom)

	Not worrisome	Somewhat worrisome	Worrisome	Very worrisome
8. Trouble breathing	1	2	3	4
9. Tired or fatigued	1	2	3	4
10. Sudden weight gain	1	2	3	4
11. Swelling	1	2	3	4
12. Dizziness, loss of balance, or passing out	1	2	3	4
13. Trouble sleeping because of trouble breathing	1	2	3	4
14. Just didn't feel well	1	2	3	4

(continued)

FIGURE 6.7

Many patients have symptoms due to their heart failure. *Trouble breathing* is the most common symptom of heart failure.

15. In the past three months, have you had trouble breathing? Circle *one*.
    1) No   2) Yes

SECTION C: *If you have NOT had trouble breathing in the last 3 months, SKIP 16–18 AND GO TO SECTION D.*

16. The *LAST TIME* you had trouble breathing, how quickly or easily did you recognize it as a symptom of heart failure? Circle *one*.
    1) I didn't
    2) It took me a while
    3) Fairly quickly
    4) Immediately

17. The *LAST FEW TIMES* you had trouble breathing, what did you do to relieve it? Circle *ALL* that apply.
    1) Reduced the sodium (salt) in your diet
    2) Reduced your fluid intake
    3) Took an extra water pill
    4) None of the above

18. **IF YOU TRIED** reducing salt in your diet, reducing your fluid intake, or taking an extra water pill, did any of these things help relieve your trouble breathing? Circle *one*.
    1) No, it did not help
    2) Yes, it helped
    3) I'm not sure if anything helped

SECTION D:

	Not confident	Somewhat confident	Very confident	Extremely confident
19. How confident are you that you can *evaluate* your symptoms?	1	2	3	4
20. Generally, how confident are you that you can *recognize changes* in your health if they occur?	1	2	3	4
21. Generally, how confident are you that you can *do something* to relieve your symptoms?	1	2	3	4
22. How confident are you that you can *evaluate the effectiveness* of whatever you do to relieve your symptoms?	1	2	3	4

Please fill in the date you completed this survey_____

Did someone help you complete this survey?   ☐ Yes   ☐ No

Source: © Barbara Riegel, 2001.

FIGURE 6.7   *(continued)*

Errors can occur at each of these stages—for example, SM strategies incorrectly matched with the problem. If a symptom has not been experienced, all of the questions related to it are skipped. Two of six symptoms must have been experienced for these subscales to be calculated; otherwise, scores may be deflated artificially. No summary score is computed because of the skip patterns in the instrument design. This instrument remains at an early stage of development.

Content validity was assessed with nurse experts and patients. Six subscales correspond to the four stages, the patient's ease in evaluating signs and symptoms, and SE. Measure of internal consistency ranged from .79 to .92. A parallel follow-up form for evaluating change over time is available from the authors. Although intended to be a self-report tool taking 15–20 minutes, some of the patients for whom it is intended may have difficulty completing it by themselves (Riegel, Carlson, Glaser, 2000). More experienced patients scored differently on the instruments, limiting their sodium intake and increasing their diuretic dose with a sudden weight gain, as would be expected (Carlson, Riegel, Moser, 2001).

References

Hypertension

Ashida, T., Sugiyama, T., Okuno, S., Ebihara, A., Fujii, J. (2000). Relationship between home blood pressure measurement and medication compliance and name recognition of antihypertensive drugs. *Hypertension Research 23*, 21–24.

Asmar, R., Zanchetti, A. (2000). Guidelines for the use of self-blood pressure monitoring: A summary report of the first international consensus conference. *Journal of Hypertension 18*, 493–508.

Boulware, L. E., et al. (2001). An evidence-based review of patient-centered behavioral interventions for hypertension. *American Journal of Preventive Medicine 23*, 221–232.

Brook, R. D. (2000). Home blood pressure: Accuracy is independent of monitoring schedules. *American Journal of Hypertension 13*, 625–631.

Campbell, N. R. C., Milkovich, L., Burgess, E., McKay, D. W. (2001). Self-measurement of blood pressure: Accuracy, patient preparation for readings, technique and equipment. *Blood Pressure Monitoring 6*, 133–138.

Denolle, T., et al. (2000). Self-measurement of blood pressure in clinical trials and therapeutic applications. *Blood Pressure Monitoring 5*, 145–149.

Jones, D. W., Hall, J. E. (2002). The National High Blood Pressure Education Program; Thirty years and counting. *Hypertension 39*, 941–942.

Masding, M. G., Jones, J. R., Bartley, E., Sandeman, D. D. (2001). Assessment of blood pressure in patients with type 2 diabetes: Comparison between home blood pressure monitoring, clinic blood pressure measurement and 24-h ambulatory blood pressure monitoring. *Diabetic Medicine 18*, 431–437.

O'Brien, E., Beevers, G., Lip, G. Y. H. (2001). Blood pressure measurement, Part IV—Automated sphygmomanometry: Self blood pressure measurement. *British Medical Journal 322*, 531–536.

Vidt, D. G. (2001). Current treatment of hypertension. *Minerva Medica 92*, 213–225.

Wilson, R. P., et al. (2002). Lay beliefs about high blood pressure in a low- to middle-income urban African-American community: An opportunity for improving hypertension control. *American Journal of Medicine 112*, 26–30.

Zarnke, K. B., Feagan, B. G., Mahon, J. L., Feldman, R. D. (1997). A randomized study comparing a patient-directed hypertension management strategy with usual office-based care. *American Journal of Hypertension 10*, 58–67.

Stroke

Boult, C., Brummel-Smith, K. (1997). Post-stroke rehabilitation guidelines. *Journal of the American Geriatric Society 45*, 881–883.

Johnson, J., Pearson, V. (2000). The effects of a structured education course on stroke survivors living in the community. *Rehabilitation Nursing 25*, 59–64.

Ottenbacher, K. J., et al. (2001). Characteristics of persons rehospitalized after stroke rehabilitation. *Archives of Physical Medicine and Rehabilitation 82*, 1367–1374.

Robinson-Smith, G. (2002). Self-efficacy and quality of life after stroke. *Journal of Neuroscience Nursing 34*, 91–98.

Anticoagulation

Christensen, T. D., Attermann, J., Hjortdal, V. E., Maegaard, M., Hasenkam, J. M. (2001). Self-management of oral anticoagulation in children with congenital heart disease. *Cardiology in the Young 11*, 269–276.

Cromheecke, M. E., et al. (2000). Oral anticoagulation self-management and management by a specialist anticoagulation clinic: A randomised cross-over comparison. *The Lancet 356*, 97–102.

Estrada, C. A., Hryniewicz, M. M., Higgs, V. B., Collins, C. B., Byrd, J. C. (2000). Anticoagulant patients information material is written at high readability levels. *Stroke 31*, 2966–2970.

Fitzmaurice, D. A., Machin, S. J. (2001). Recommendations for patients undertaking self management of oral anticoagulation. *British Medical Journal 323*, 985–989.

Koertke, H., Minami, K., Bairaktaris, A., Wagner, O., Koerfer, R. (2000). INR self-management following mechanical heart valve replacement. *Journal of Thrombosis and Thrombolysis 9*, S41–S45.

Morsdorf, S., et al. (1999). Training of patients for self-management of oral anticoagulant therapy: Standards, patient suitability, and clinical aspects. *Seminars in Thrombosis and Hemostasis 25*, 109–115.

Sidhu, P., O'Kane, H. O. (2001). Self-managed anticoagulation: Results from a two-year prospective randomized trial with heart valve patients. *Annals of Thoracic Surgery 72*, 1523–1527.

Taborski, U., Muller-Berghaus, G. (1999). State-of-the-art patient self-management for control of oral anticoagulation. *Seminars in Thrombosis and Hemostasis 25*, 43–47.

Heart Failure

Ahmed, A. (2002). Quality and outcomes of heart failure care in older adults: Role of multidisciplinary disease-management programs. *Journal of the American Geriatrics Society 50*, 1590–1593.

Bennett, S. J., Cordes, D. K., Westmoreland, G., Castro, R., Donnelly, E. (2000). Self-care strategies for symptom management in patients with chronic heart failure. *Nursing Research 49*, 139–145.

Blue, L., et al. (2001). Randomised controlled trial of specialist nurse intervention in heart failure. *British Medical Journal 323*, 715–718.

Carlson, B., Riegel, B., Moser, D. K. (2001). Self-care abilities of patients with heart failure. *Heart & Lung 30*, 351–359.

Cline, C. M. J., Israelsson, B. Y. A., Willenheimer, R. B., Broms, K., Erhardt, L. R. (1998). Cost effective management programme for heart failure reduces hospitalisation. *Heart 80*, 442–446.

Dunbar, S. B., Jacobson, L. H., Deaton, C. (1998). Heart failure: Strategies to enhance patient self-management. *AACN Clinical Issues 9*, 244–256.

Fonarow, G. C., et al. (1997). Impact of a comprehensive heart failure management program on hospital readmission and functional status of patients with advanced heart failure. *Journal of the American Geriatric Association 30,* 725–732.

Harrison, M. B., et al. (2002). Quality of life of individuals with heart failure. *Medical Care 40,* 271–282.

Moser, D. K. (2000). Heart failure management: Optimal health care delivery programs. *Annual Review of Nursing Research 18,* 91–126.

Rich, M. W. (1999). Heart failure disease management: A critical review. *Journal of Cardiac Failure 5,* 64–75.

Riegel, B., et al. (2002a). Effect of a standardized nurse case-management telephone intervention on resource use in patients with chronic heart failure. *Archives of Internal Medicine 162,* 705–712.

Riegel, B., et al. (2002b). Cognitive impairment in heart failure: Issues of measurement and etiology. *American Journal of Critical Care 11,* 520–528.

Riegel, B., Carlson, B., Glaser, D. (2000). Development and testing of a clinical tool measuring self-management of heart failure. *Heart & Lung 29,* 4–12.

7

Self-Management Preparation for Other Diseases

 Some disease entities for which SM are very appropriate have never developed this tradition or, in the case of renal replacement therapy, abandoned it after policy changes made SM fiscally unrewarding for providers. Although the SM literature in these areas is miniscule, this fact does not necessarily mean that patients would not benefit from an opportunity to do SM and to be prepared for it.

End-Stage Renal Disease/Renal Replacement Therapy Self-Management Preparation

End-stage renal disease (ESRD) currently affects more than 340,000 U.S. residents, 60% of whom are treated with hemodialysis (Welch, 2001). Most ESRD patients are covered by Medicare; the total cost of this care in 1998 was $12 billion — serving 0.7% of the Medicare population, but consuming 5% of the annual Medicare budget (Xue, Ma, Louis, Collins, 2001). An important distinction can be made in the degree of patient involvement in the delivery of the different forms of dialysis. Center hemodialysis is performed three times per week by nurses or technicians. Some patients dialyze at home and are able to set and maintain their own hemodialysis schedules. Continuous ambulatory peritoneal dialysis (CAPD) requires patients to take an even more active role (Christensen, Ehlers, 2002).

Renal replacement therapy (RRT) presents an interesting case example of a field that began with nearly universal SM and was almost entirely reversed through payment policies to become provided services. Begun in 1961, home hemodialysis expanded in the 1970s (39% of patients dialyzed at home in 1972) and early 1980s. By 1992, only 1.3% dialyzed at home, even though this modality offers higher quality of life, more independence, and better rehabilitation, in part because treatment schedule can be individualized to patient need. It is also less expensive. Home hemodialysis is, however, restricted to patients with no major medical contraindications, good vascular access, and room and assistance in their homes (Mackenzie, Mactier, 1998). Similar patterns have been found in Europe (Feraud, Wauters, 1999). Current patterns of center dialysis may be unsustainable because of costs.

Currently, many new ESRD patients are elderly and have diabetes; home hemodialysis is more difficult for them and their helpers are also frequently elderly (unless paid helpers are used). The trend toward provided services for ESRD patients is now beginning to reverse in part because of increasing interest in use of more frequent dialysis. After adjustment for patient case mix and comorbidity, persons on home hemodialysis have improved quality of life, independence, and rehabilitation in comparison with other dialysis modalities (Mackenzie, Mactier, 1998).

Blagg (2000) explains that the initial payments to facilities for center dialysis were generous while the payments for home hemodialysis were inadequate, with some supplies not being covered. Fees paid for home training were insufficient, and the three-month waiting period for patients to become Medicare-entitled meant that they could not start on home hemodialysis until the waiting period ended. Physicians were not paid for supervision of patient training, and for-profit dialysis units did not provide or support home dialysis. Although Medicare regulations currently require all patients be given the option to select home hemodialysis or transplantation, few dialysis units currently train patients to do so. Those few facilities that do train them to track and maintain dialysis adequacy, access care, monitor lab values, use clinic procedures for emergencies, and understand patient rights and responsbilities.

In the late 1970s, continuous ambulatory peritoneal dialysis, which has a short training time, filled the needs of many patients. Twenty-eight percent of ESRD patients have a functioning transplant and are responsible for management of their immunosuppressive regimen, having lab tests done, and monitoring themselves for early signs of rejection or infection (Christensen, Ehlers, 2002).

Currently, education for pre-ESRD patients is proving beneficial. Begun when creatinine clearance is at 30 mL/min, such education has been shown to allow a greater number of blue-collar workers to remain employed after starting dialysis, to decrease incidence of emergency dialysis compared with control patients, and to start dialysis as an outpatient rather than in hospital (Golper, 2001).

Multiple Sclerosis Self-Management Preparation

Multiple Sclerosis (MS) is the most common chronic and unpredictable neurological disease affecting young and middle-aged adults. It appears in more than twice as many women as men, with peak onset at 33 years. MS causes demyelinization of the central nervous system (CNS), resulting in delayed or blocked transmission of nerve impulses. Because any of the myelinated fibers in the CNS may be damaged by MS, the variety of problems caused by the disease is wide-ranging: abnormal gait, bladder and bowel problems, visual and speech disturbances, memory problems, and fatigue. Its course is variable (Shnek, Foley, LaRocca, Smith, Halper, 1995).

Standards for Self-Management Preparation
None could be located.

Effective Interventions and Measurement Instruments

Learning may be affected by cognitive distortions, including catastrophizing, overgeneralization, personalization, and selective abstraction.

A primary focus of MS SM is symptom management. For example, the fatigue of MS comes on quickly, more frequently, and with greater severity and requires a much longer recovery period than does normal fatigue; it also seems to exacerbate other symptoms. A RCT of an energy conservation course for individuals with fatigue secondary to MS (Mathiowetz, Matuska, Murphy, 2001) found the experimental group with less fatigue, increased SE, and improved quality of life in comparison with a control group.

The MS Beliefs Scale (a measure of SE) (Shnek, Foley, LaRocca, Smith, Halper, 1995) is the same as the Arthritis Beliefs Scale, but with the wording changed to MS. Depressed MS patients were likely to report lower SE than were patients who were not depressed. No other validity checks of this instrument for a MS population could be found — important because validity for an arthritis population cannot be assumed for a different population.

The MS Self-Efficacy Scale (MSSE) (Schwartz, Coulthard-Morris, Zeng, Retzlaff, 1996) appears in Figure 7.1. This instrument emulates the format of the Arthritis SE Scale but with additional items reflecting symptoms appropriate to MS. Scores for the three subscales are obtained by summing item scores. Confirmatory factor analysis showed two subscales: SE function, which measures sense of confidence to perform daily living activities (alpha, .86; test-retest, .81), and SE control, which measures confidence in one's disease-related limitations and the disease's effects on life activities (alpha, .90; test-retest, .62). The overall instrument had an alpha of .89 and test-retest reliability of .75. The SE function subscale's association with actual functional limitations is consistent with convergent validity.

HIV/AIDS Self-Management Preparation

With early detection and effective care, many of the 1 million Americans thought to be infected with HIV can expect to live full, productive lives for decades; thus a chronic disease model

The Multiple Sclerosis Self-Efficacy Scale (MSSE)

	Very uncertain			Moderately certain			Very certain		

FUNCTION: *As of now, how certain are you that you can:*

1. Walk 100 feet on flat ground?	10	20	30	40	50	60	70	80	90	100
2. Walk 10 steps downstairs?	10	20	30	40	50	60	70	80	90	100
3. Take good care of your home or yard?	10	20	30	40	50	60	70	80	90	100
4. Get dressed or undressed without assistance?	10	20	30	40	50	60	70	80	90	100
5. Get in and out of the passenger side of a car without assistance from another person and without physical aids?	10	20	30	40	50	60	70	80	90	100
6. Speak clearly to express your needs or ideas?	10	20	30	40	50	60	70	80	90	100
7. Write clearly so that others can read what you wrote?	10	20	30	40	50	60	70	80	90	100
8. Take a bath or shower without assistance from someone else?	10	20	30	40	50	60	70	80	90	100
9. Go on a trip that keeps you away from home for the whole day?	10	20	30	40	50	60	70	80	90	100

CONTROL

1. How certain are you that you can control your fatigue?	10	20	30	40	50	60	70	80	90	100
2. How certain are you that you can regulate your activity so as to be active without aggravating your MS?	10	20	30	40	50	60	70	80	90	100
3. As compared to other people with MS like yours, how certain are you that you can manage your MS symptoms during your daily activities?	10	20	30	40	50	60	70	80	90	100
4. How certain are you that you can manage your MS symptoms so that you can do the things you enjoy doing?	10	20	30	40	50	60	70	80	90	100
5. How certain are you that you can deal with the frustration of MS?	10	20	30	40	50	60	70	80	90	100
6. How certain are you that you can deal with the uncertainty of MS?	10	20	30	40	50	60	70	80	90	100
7. How certain are you that you can decrease your fatigue quite a bit?	10	20	30	40	50	60	70	80	90	100
8. How certain are you that you can continue most of your daily activities?	10	20	30	40	50	60	70	80	90	100
9. How certain are you that you can keep your MS symptoms from interfering with your time spent with friends or family?	10	20	30	40	50	60	70	80	90	100

Source: Schwartz, C. E., Coulthard-Morris, L., Zeng, Q., Retzlaff, P. (1996). Measuring self-efficacy in people with multiple sclerosis: A validation study. *Archives of Physical Medicine and Rehabilitation 77*, 394–398. Reprinted with permission from The American Congress of Rehabilitation Medicine and The American Academy of Physical Medicine and Rehabilitation.

FIGURE 7.1

including SM is relevant for this disease. The pharmacologic agents used in treating this disease improve immune status and prolong life by reducing viral load but can also cause side effects. If they are not taken reliably, drug resistance may develop rapidly. For these reasons, side effects that could interfere with taking the medication must be resolved and skills to manage the regimen itself must be assured. Clearly, HIV patients must be competent participants in their own care (Gifford, Sengupta, 1999).

Persons with AIDS must manage multiple symptoms, follow a very complex regimen, and deal with social stigma. Because the disease frequently involves neuropsychiatric symptoms, including confusion, and disproportionately affects the poor, who may have limited learning skills, the ability to learn and retain SM skills may be problematic. In addition, HIV patients are often IV drug users and racial/ethnic minorities who may have difficulty in accessing health and social services and, therefore, need substantial education and support (Gifford, Sengupta, 1999).

Standards for Self-Management Preparation
None could be located.

Effective Interventions and Measurement Instruments
Three well-developed examples of HIV/AIDS SM preparation studied through rigorous research designs are discussed to show commonalities in approach and effectiveness.

Gifford and colleagues (Gifford, Laurent, Gonzales, Chesney, Lorig, 1998; Gifford, Sengupta, 1999) taught symptomatic HIV/AIDS patients to self-manage what is frequently a complicated medication regimen, to interpret and act on symptoms, and to engage in physical exercise, relaxation, doctor–patient communication, nutrition, and motivation. This Positive Self-Management Program (PSMP) was structured to include setting and achieving goals, by using patient–caregiver descriptions of the problems of living with HIV, including unrecognized problems of fatigue, depression, helplessness, and barriers encountered in solving the problems. Patients were taught how to respond appropriately to new symptoms, which might be dangerous and require urgent attention. They were also taught how to function with neuropathy-related paresthesias and generalized fatigue, depression, anger, and stress.

Seven weekly sessions were held. Group instruction was led by trained peer-leaders, one of whom had HIV infection and tried to model coping behaviors and enhance SE. Many long-term caregivers of people with HIV/AIDS have also been leaders. Instruction was accommodated to expressed needs and concerns of patients and was directed by a leader manual and a patient resource book. Groups were closed to maximize confidentiality and group cohesion. They met in community settings such as churches or clinics, located conveniently to participants' homes and to public transportation.

Contracting was used to enhance a sense of performance accomplishment, which also leads to increased SE. Each week members reported on their contracts to the group and received immediate feedback on any problems encountered. Vicarious experiences raise efficacy perceptions by allowing individuals to see others succeeding at important tasks.

Three months post-intervention, the symptom severity index (number of symptoms of moderate or greater severity) decreased in the experimental group and increased in the control group, which had received the usual medical care; the same was true for SE for controlling symptoms. No significant differences between the groups were found for pain, fatigue, and psychological symptoms. These studies were done with relatively well-educated male participants.

A second rigorous model was studied by Inouye, Flannelly, and Flannelly (2001). This program focused on SM preparation and particularly on coping skills training, which has become a central element of treatment intervention programs. The majority of studies of behavioral-cognitive treatment have reported a decrease in depression and stress, although they have not found any immunological effects. This program provided seven weeks of biofeedback for relaxation; cognitive-behavioral treatment for anxiety, anger, and depression; and educational materials and problem-solving practice. In comparison with a control group, coping strategies in the SM group were significantly improved, with an increase in mood and a decrease in anger, confusion, tension, depression, and fatigue. SM training significantly decreased use of emotive, fatalistic, and palliative coping styles relative to controls.

Finally, Leenerts and Magilvy (2000) studied the experience of self-care in low-income, HIV-positive white women. Histories of abuse were common, damaging their self-images and leaving the patients disconnected from self-care. The shock of the diagnosis left these women estranged from their bodies and their self-care. Those who were treated with disregard and disparagement at the time of diagnosis disconnected from the health care system, in some cases for as long as 18 months. Upon entering the health care system, they were often uncertain and even confused about what they needed to live with HIV infection. Outreach efforts were critical to finding these women and bringing them to health care.

The experience of being cared for provided an important catalyst for motivation to learn and engage in self-care and SM practices. Investment in SM took place over time and was accelerated by important turning points, such as pregnancy and childbirth, death of loved ones, substance abuse, and mental health treatment. All participants expressed concern about their ability to communicate their own needs and make themselves understood by health care providers and significant others.

These women were socialized to identify care as self-sacrifice and to inhibit self-expression and action so as to protect relationships. The fear of disconnection from relationships — even abusive ones — kept their attention diverted from SM. Women's groups and shelters with role models and self-care examples were important to repairing a damaged sense of self.

These three examples of SM preparation for persons with HIV/AIDS share several characteristics: structured educational programs, a focus on coping, and the experience of learning and practicing SM.

Two studies (Kalichman, Ramachandran, Catz, 1999; Kalichman, Rompa, 2000) showed that persons of low literacy were more likely to miss treatment doses because of confusion, depression, and desire to cleanse their bodies than were participants with higher health literacy. Indeed, education and health literacy levels were significant and independent predictors of treatment adherence. HIV-infected individuals with lower health literacy had lower CD4 cell counts, had higher viral loads, were less likely to be taking antiretroviral medications, and reported a greater number of hospitalizations and poorer health than did those with higher health literacy. In these studies, about one of four persons living with HIV/AIDS demonstrated difficulty comprehending simple medical instructions, making health literacy a significant factor in the health and treatment of persons living with this disease.

People of lower literacy may benefit from pictorial displays of their medications, accurate in color and size, with graphic illustration of the instructions, including the number of pills to be taken and the times at which to take them. In addition, videotapes tailored to different levels of comprehension will provide a more effective communication medium than pamphlets and brochures for educating patients about their treatments. Low education and low literacy suggest the importance of including concrete practices with lots of repetition and follow-up.

No measurement instruments concerning SM preparation were located.

Epilepsy Self-Management Preparation

Although epilepsy is a serious disease with much opportunity for life disruption, SM preparation is not standard for it. Concern for the quality of epilepsy care has been most pronounced in the United Kingdom; several surveys have identified even basic provision of information to patients as poor, particularly for the elderly. Patients perceive their general practitioners — and many GPs perceive themselves — as having a limited knowledge of epilepsy (Poole et al., 2000).

Incorrect information is common. In one study of adults, 30% believed that epilepsy is a mental disorder or contagious, and 25% that pregnant women with epilepsy should discontinue their antiepilepsy drugs (AEDs) to prevent teratogenic side effects (Long, Reeves, Moore, Roach, Pickering, 2000).

Sixty to ninety percent of persons with epilepsy can achieve a remission in seizures (Kwan, Ridsdale, Robins, 2000). In the special population of adults with learning disabilities, 20% had at least one seizure per year, with half of individuals with severe or profound learning disability having epilepsy (Clark, Espie, Paul, 2001).

Seizures are the most frequently occurring neurological condition in children. Three to five percent of all children experience seizures, and 10% to 20% of children who experience them in infancy or early childhood will experience them recurrently. A limited body of longitudinal research provides limited guidance about the medical and developmental trajectories of children with early-onset seizures or the process of coping and adaptation in families. Parents commonly indicated need for information about the effects of seizures on their child's early development and learning, such as how they affect the brain. Parents also wanted information on what to do when a child has a seizure, and they needed educational materials that could be shared with relatives, child care providers, and teachers. Many parents feel medical professionals devote inadequate time and attention to family and emotional issues related to coping with seizures (Aytch, Hammond, White, 2001).

The significant stigma experienced by children with epilepsy as compared with those with asthma or diabetes has been described by Houston, Cunningham, Metcalfe, and Newton (2000). The five- to ten-year-olds with epilepsy that the researchers studied had far more questions, felt excluded from discussions with doctors, and appeared reluctant to tell friends about their diagnosis. In comparison with children with either diabetes or asthma, those with epilepsy reported experiencing more psychosocial problems, including feelings of being less happy, less valuable, and less successful than others, being more likely to be teased, feeling isolated, and finding it difficult to integrate into school and community life.

When compared with children with better-controlled seizures, those with less well-controlled epilepsy exhibited a poorer self-image, more depression, lower perceived competence, more irritability, and more social withdrawal. Half of parents reported that their child experienced seizure medication side effects, including confusion, sleepiness, irritability, aggressiveness, slurred speech, poor balance, and marked sleep disruption (Aytch, Hammond, White, 2001). Similar problems and lack of accurate information may be found among youth with epilepsy, who also are known to have high rates of mental health problems including poor self-esteem, depression, and behavior problems (Austin, McNelis, Shore, Dunn, Musick, 2002).

Epilepsy SM has been defined as activities that an individual can perform alone and that are known to either control the frequency of seizures or promote the well-being of the person with seizures (Dilorio, Faherty, Manteuffel, 1992a). It includes taking AEDs, employing behavioral techniques to decrease seizure frequency, and making adjustments in lifestyle to control seizures and foster physical safety. Patients must also understand diagnostic tests such as EEGs and MRIs, effects of AEDs on family planning, safety regarding driving and use of some equipment, and legal restrictions on jobs such as firefighting, heavy goods handling, and vehicle driving. Safety precautions include not using power tools, not swimming alone, and not climbing on high ladders. Caregivers must know first-aid seizure care (Kwan, Ridsdale, Robins, 2000).

Individuals with frequent attacks should keep a seizure diary, charting the times and dates of seizures and administration of medications, presence of an aura, or specific preceding triggers. It may be possible to recognize factors that precipitate the seizures, such as stress levels, too much alcohol, excessive heat or cold environments, or flashing strobe lights (Kwan, Ridsdale, Robins, 2000). Some people can prevent seizures by using distraction when they feel one is imminent or can stop seizures in evolution or control them through use of relaxation, self-hypnosis, and stress management. Seizure calendars are useful in determining adequacy of medications (Dilorio, Henry, 1995).

Standards for Self-Management Preparation
None could be located.

Effective Interventions and Measurement Instruments

Tieffenberg, Wood, Alonso, Tossutti, and Vincente (2000) report on a school-based training model for children with chronic illnesses including epilepsy, relying on play and coordinated by teachers. Five weekly meetings of eight to ten families were held simultaneously with children's and parent's groups. Children in the experimental group showed positive changes in school absenteeism and decreased numbers of seizures and emergency and routine health care visits.

German authors (May, Pfafflin, 2002) report development of an epilepsy patient education program called Modular Service Package Epilepsy (MOSES). It includes 14 lessons lasting 60 minutes each on the following topics: living with epilepsy, epidemiology, basic knowledge, diagnostics, therapy, self-control, prognosis, psychosocial aspects, and networking. MOSES has been tested in a RCT, where participants showed significantly fewer seizures and more knowledge, satisfaction, and coping skills as compared with a control group. MOSES does not appear to be focused primarily on SM preparation.

Dilorio and colleagues have developed both the Epilepsy Self-Management Scale (ESMS; Figure 7.2) and the Epilepsy Self-Efficacy Scale (ESES; Figure 7.3) (Dilorio, Faherty, Manteuffel, 1992a, 1992b; Dilorio, Henry, 1995). Content validity was based on discussions with people with epilepsy and their health professionals. The measure of internal consistency for ESMS was .86. Score is the sum of individual items. Scores may range from 36 to 180, with higher scores indicating more frequent use of SM strategies. The ESES assesses confidence in performing tasks related to medication taking, seizure control, and general epilepsy SM. Content validity was reviewed by an expert panel. Internal consistency reliability was .93 and test-retest reliability was .81. Possible scores range from 0 to 2500. A strong positive correlation between SE and SM supported construct validity.

The Epilepsy Knowledge Scale (EKS) was used in the evaluation of an educational program intended to improve patients' knowledge and understanding of their epilepsy. These outcomes are necessary but not sufficient for SM. The EKS's internal consistency reliability was .72. Scores ranged from 0 to 100 (May, Pfafflin, 2002).

Epilepsy Self-Management Scale (ESMS)

	Never		Always
If I am going to be away from home, I take my seizure medication with me.	1	...	5

When the doctor orders blood tests, I have them done.

If I had side effects from the seizure medication, I would skip a dose without asking my doctor.*

I take my seizure medication the way the doctor orders it.

I drink a lot of alcoholic beverages such as beer, wine, and whiskey.*

When my seizure medication is running out, I take less medication at each time.*

I have to put off having my seizure medication refilled because it costs too much money.*

I miss doctor or clinic appointments.*

I plan ahead and have my seizure medication refilled before I run out.

I skip doses of seizure medication.*

I call my doctor if I am having more seizures than usual.

I use power tools such as electric saws, electric hedge trimmers, or electric knives.*

I take my seizure medication at the same time each day.

I stay out of situations that might cause a seizure.

I miss doses of my seizure medication because I do not remember to take it.*

I stay away from things that make me have seizures.

I would go swimming alone.*

I make sure I get enough sleep.

I stay out late at night.*

I eat regular meals.

I have a way to remind myself to take my seizure medication.

I think positive thoughts.

I check with my doctor before taking other medicines.

I climb objects such as high stools, chairs, or ladders.*

I call my doctor when I think I am having side effects from my seizure medication.

I wear or carry information stating that I have epilepsy.

I talk with other people who have epilepsy.

I keep track of the side effects of my seizure medication.

I keep a record of when my seizures have occurred.

I keep a record of the types of seizures I have.

I use relaxation techniques to keep myself from having a seizure.

I write down the number of seizures I have.

I use guided imagery to keep myself from having a seizure.

I participate in a support group for persons with epilepsy.

I use self-hypnosis to keep myself from having a seizure.

*These items were recorded so that higher scores reflect more positive self-management practices.

Source: Dilorio, C., Henry, M. (1995). Self-management in persons with epilepsy. *Journal of Neuroscience Nursing* 27, 338–343. Reprinted with permission from the American Association of Neuroscience Nurses.

FIGURE 7.2

Epilepsy Self-Efficacy Scale

	I cannot do at all				Moderately sure I can do					Sure I can do	
1. I can always take my seizure medication when I am away from home.	0	1	2	3	4	5	6	7	8	9	10
2. I can stay on my seizure medication most of the time.	0	1	2	3	4	5	6	7	8	9	10
*3. I can always practice relaxation exercises to help me manage stress.	0	1	2	3	4	5	6	7	8	9	10
4. I can always name my seizure medication.	0	1	2	3	4	5	6	7	8	9	10
5. I can always plan ahead so that I do not run out of my seizure medication.	0	1	2	3	4	5	6	7	8	9	10
*6. I can always get enough exercise.	0	1	2	3	4	5	6	7	8	9	10
7. I can always take my seizure medication on holidays, birthdays, vacations, and other special occasions.	0	1	2	3	4	5	6	7	8	9	10
8. I can have fun with other people and still manage my epilepsy.	0	1	2	3	4	5	6	7	8	9	10
9. I can always take my seizure medication around people who do not know that I have seizures.	0	1	2	3	4	5	6	7	8	9	10
*10. I can always use stress management techniques to stop seizures.	0	1	2	3	4	5	6	7	8	9	10
11. I can always take care of day-to-day changes in my epilepsy.	0	1	2	3	4	5	6	7	8	9	10
12. I can always manage my epilepsy in new situations.	0	1	2	3	4	5	6	7	8	9	10
13. I can always tell when I am having side effects from my seizure medication.	0	1	2	3	4	5	6	7	8	9	10
*14. I can always eat healthy meals.	0	1	2	3	4	5	6	7	8	9	10
15. I can always deal with any side effects from my seizure medication.	0	1	2	3	4	5	6	7	8	9	10
16. I can always manage my epilepsy.	0	1	2	3	4	5	6	7	8	9	10
*17. I can always recognize situations or activities that may make my seizures worse.	0	1	2	3	4	5	6	7	8	9	10
18. I can always find ways to get enough sleep.	0	1	2	3	4	5	6	7	8	9	10
19. I can always handle situations that upset me.	0	1	2	3	4	5	6	7	8	9	10
20. I can always fit my seizure medication schedule around my daily activities.	0	1	2	3	4	5	6	7	8	9	10
21. I can always do what needs to be done if I miss a dose of my seizure medication.	0	1	2	3	4	5	6	7	8	9	10

FIGURE 7.3

	I cannot do at all				Moderately sure I can do				Sure I can do	
*22. I can always find ways to do things that I enjoy to help me manage stress.	0	1	2	3	4	5	6	7	8	9	10
23. I can always follow my seizure medication schedule.	0	1	2	3	4	5	6	7	8	9	10
24. I can always call my doctor or nurse when I need to ask a question or report a seizure.	0	1	2	3	4	5	6	7	8	9	10
25. I can always keep my epilepsy under control.	0	1	2	3	4	5	6	7	8	9	10
26. I can always take time out from my daily activities to go to the doctor for an epilepsy check-up.	0	1	2	3	4	5	6	7	8	9	10
*27. I can always avoid situations or activities that make my seizures worse.	0	1	2	3	4	5	6	7	8	9	10
28. I can always drive or get a ride to the doctor's office when I need to see him or her.	0	1	2	3	4	5	6	7	8	9	10
29. I can always get medical help when needed for my seizures.	0	1	2	3	4	5	6	7	8	9	10
30. I can always find ways to remember to take my seizure medication.	0	1	2	3	4	5	6	7	8	9	10
*31. I always carry personal identification in case I have a seizure.	0	1	2	3	4	5	6	7	8	9	10
32. I can always find a way to get seizure medication if I go out of town and forget mine.	0	1	2	3	4	5	6	7	8	9	10
33. I can always get my seizure medication refilled when I need to.	0	1	2	3	4	5	6	7	8	9	10

*Items added for ESES 2000.

Source: Dilorio, C., Yeager, K. (2003). The Epilepsy Self-Efficacy Scale. In Strickland, O. L., Dilorio, C. (Eds). *Measurement of Nursing Outcomes: Self Care and Coping.* Vol. 3 (2nd ed.), pp. 40–51. New York: Springer Publishing Company. Reprinted with permission from the author.

FIGURE 7.3 *(continued)*

Knowledge scales exist for all other chronic diseases and may be found in Redman (2003). They are not included in this book because knowledge is a basic prerequisite for SM but never sufficient. Because many individuals with epilepsy apparently are not provided with access to this basic prerequisite, EKS is included here (Figure 7.4).

Epilepsy Knowledge Scale (EKS), Parts I and II

Part	Questions	Yes	No	I Do Not Know
I	People with epilepsy should avoid strenuous work because it can provoke seizures.	☐	■	☐
	An EEG can always prove the diagnosis of epilepsy.	☐	■	☐
	People with epilepsy are as capable as other people.	■	☐	☐
	All people with seizures should avoid working with open machinery.	☐	■	☐
	Every seizure destroys a number of nerve cells in the brain.	☐	■	☐
	People with seizures should not swim without an accompanying person.	■	☐	☐
	All people with epilepsy should avoid flashing or strobing lights (e.g., disco lights, TV or computer screens).	☐	■	☐
	In most cases, doctors can control epileptic seizures with medication.	■	☐	☐
	If your seizures are controlled for some months, you can reduce the dose of antiepileptic medication.	☐	■	☐
II	All people with epilepsy have similar symptoms.	☐	■	☐
	If a patient expects a seizure, he or she should take an additional dose of antiepileptic medication.	☐	■	☐
	On a job application, a patient should always disclose his or her epilepsy condition.	☐	■	☐
	People with epilepsy can take an active part in sports.	■	☐	☐
	An epileptic seizure always results in loss of consciousness.	☐	■	☐
	People whose seizures happen only during sleep may hold a driver's license.	■	☐	☐
	Everyone can have a seizure, given the appropriate circumstances.	■	☐	☐
	Blood samples can be used to measure the concentration of antiepileptic medication in the body.	■	☐	☐
	Epilepsy is a symptom of mental illness.	☐	■	☐
	If persons with epilepsy drive, they must inform the driving authorities about their condition.	☐	■	☐

■ Correct answer.

Source: May, T. W., Pfafflin, M. (2002). The efficacy of an educational treatment program for patients with epilepsy (MOSES): Results of a controlled, randomized study. *Epilepsia 43*, 539–549.

FIGURE 7.4

In the United Kingdom, the role of a nurse specialist in epilepsy is emerging as a force, just as it has for persons with diabetes and asthma. These nurses monitor treatment, provide advice, offer SM preparation, and act as liaisons with other health professionals (Kwan, Ridsdale, Robins, 2000).

References

End-Stage Renal Disease/Renal Replacement Therapy

Blagg, C. (2000). What went wrong with home hemodialysis in the United States and what can be done now? *Hemodialysis International 4,* 55–57.

Christensen, A. J., Ehlers, S. L. (2002). Psychological factors in end-stage renal disease: An emerging context for behavioral medicine research. *Journal of Consulting and Clinical Psychology 70,* 712–724.

Feraud, P., Wauters, J. (1999). The decline of home hemodialysis: How and why? *Nephron 81,* 249–255.

Golper, T. (2001). Patient education: Can it maximize the success of therapy? *Nephrology Dialysis Transplantation 16* (Suppl 7), 20–24.

Mackenzie, P., Mactier, R. A. (1998). Home haemodialysis in the 1990s. *Nephrology Dialysis Transplantation 13,* 1944–1948.

Welch, J. L. (2001). Hemodialysis patient beliefs by stage of fluid adherence. *Research in Nursing & Health 24,* 105–112.

Xue, J. L., Ma, J. Z., Louis, T. A., Collins, A. J. (2001). Forecast of the number of patients with end-stage renal disease in the United States by year 2010. *Journal of the American Society of Nephrology 12,* 2753–2758.

Multiple Sclerosis

Mathiowetz, V., Matuska, K. M., Murphy, M. E. (2001). Efficacy of an energy conservation course for persons with multiple sclerosis. *Archives of Physical Medicine and Rehabilitation 42,* 449–456.

Schwartz, C. E., Coulthard-Morris, L., Zeng, Q., Retzlaff, P. (1996). Measuring self-efficacy in people with multiple sclerosis: A validation study. *Archives of Physical Medicine and Rehabilitation 77,* 394–398.

Shnek, Z. M., Foley, F. W., LaRocca, N. G., Smith, C. R., Halper, J. (1995). Psychological predictors of depression in multiple sclerosis. *Journal of Neurological Rehabilitation 9,* 15–23.

HIV/AIDS

Gifford, A. L., Laurent, D. D., Gonzales, V. M., Chesney, M. A., Lorig, K. R. (1998). Pilot randomized trial of education to improve self-management skills of men with symptomatic HIV/AIDS. *Journal of Acquired Immune Deficiency Syndromes and Human Retrovirology 18*, 136–144.

Gifford, A. L., Sengupta, S. (1999). Self-management health education for chronic HIV infection. *AIDS Care 11*, 115–130.

Inouye, J., Flannelly, L., Flannelly, K. J. (2001). The effectiveness of self-management training for individuals with HIV/AIDS. *Journal of the Association of Nurses in AIDS Care 12(5)*, 71–82.

Kalichman, S. C., Ramachandran, B., Catz, S. (1999). Adherence to combination antiretroviral therapies in patients of low health literacy. *Journal of General Internal Medicine 14*, 267–273.

Kalichman, S. C., Rompa, D. (2000). Functional health literacy is associated with health status and health-related knowledge in people living with HIV-AIDS. *Journal of Acquired Immune Deficiency Syndromes 25*, 337–344.

Leenerts, M. H., Magilvy, J. K. (2000). Investing in self-care: A midrange theory of self-care grounded in the lived experience of low-income HIV-positive white women. *Advances in Nursing Science 22(3)*, 58–75.

Epilepsy

Austin, J. K., McNelis, A. M., Shore, C. P., Dunn, D. W., Musick, B. (2002). A feasibility study of a family seizure management program: "Be Seizure Smart." *Journal of Neuroscience Nursing 34*, 30–37.

Aytch, L. S., Hammond, R., White, C. (2001). Seizures in infants and young children: An exploratory study of family experiences and needs for information and support. *Journal of Neuroscience Nursing 33*, 278–285.

Clark, A. J., Espie, C. A., Paul, A. (2001). Adults with learning disabilities and epilepsy: Knowledge about epilepsy before and after an educational package. *Seizure 10*, 492–499.

Dilorio, C., Faherty, B., Manteuffel, B. (1992a). Self-efficacy and social support in self-management of epilepsy. *Western Journal of Nursing Research 14*, 292–307.

Dilorio, C., Faherty, B., Manteuffel, B. (1992b). The development and testing of an instrument to measure self-efficacy in individuals with epilepsy. *Journal of Neuroscience Nursing 24*, 9–13.

Dilorio, C., Henry, M. (1995). Self-management in persons with epilepsy. *Journal of Neuroscience Nursing 27,* 338–343.

Houston, E. C., Cunningham, C. C., Metcalfe, E., Newton, R. (2000). The information needs and understanding of 5–10 year old children with epilepsy, asthma or diabetes. *Seizure 9,* 340–343.

Kwan, I., Ridsdale, L., Robins, D. (2000). An epilepsy care package: The nurse specialist's role. *Journal of Neuroscience Nursing 32,* 145–152.

Long, L., Reeves, A. L., Moore, J. L., Roach, J., Pickering, C. T. (2000). An assessment of epilepsy patients' knowledge of their disorder. *Epilepsia 41,* 727–731.

May, T. W., Pfafflin, M. (2002). The efficacy of an educational treatment program for patients with epilepsy (MOSES): Results of a controlled, randomized study. *Epilepsia 34,* 539–549.

Poole, K., et al. (2000). Patients' perspectives on services for epilepsy: A survey of patient satisfaction, preferences and information provision in 2394 people with epilepsy. *Seizure 9,* 551–558.

Redman, B. K. (2003). *Measurement tools in patient education,* 2nd ed. New York, Springer Publishing.

Tieffenberg J. A., Wood, E. I., Alonso, A., Tossutti, M. S., Vincente, M. F. (2000). A randomized field trial of ACINDES: A child-centered training model for children with chronic illnesses (asthma and epilepsy). *Journal of Urban Health 77,* 280–297.

8

Asthma and Chronic Obstructive Pulmonary Disease Self-Management Preparation

Asthma Self-Management Preparation

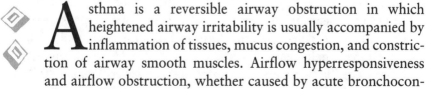

Asthma is a reversible airway obstruction in which heightened airway irritability is usually accompanied by inflammation of tissues, mucus congestion, and constriction of airway smooth muscles. Airflow hyperresponsiveness and airflow obstruction, whether caused by acute bronchoconstriction, airway edema, chronic mucus plug formation, or changes in the lung matrix, are important components of the disease. Roughly half of all patients with asthma experience not only a reaction that appears seconds after exposure and lasts about an hour, but also a delayed or late-phase reaction that begins four to eight hours after exposure and lasts for hours or days (Reinke, Hoffman, 2000). Chronic inflammation causes these patients' airways to become hyperresponsive not only to specific antigens, but also to stimuli such as physical exertion, breathing cold air, and tobacco smoke. Recovery is usually defined as movement into the normal range; small improvements can be clinically significant (Lehrer, Feldman, Giardino, Song, Schmaling, 2002).

The prevalence of asthma in North America and Europe is about 5% of the adult population and 7% of children, with strong evidence of increasing incidence. Morbidity and mortality increase disproportionately in indigent inner-city populations. A study of nearly 3000 asthma patients in health plans found that one-fourth of them experienced severe symptoms. These affected individuals were more likely to be from minority groups, women, with less than a college education, current smokers, and receiving care from nonspecialists. As compared with mild/moderate asthmatics, severe asthmatics reported having less of an understanding of the clinical manifestations of asthma and the means to manage an exacerbation (Liu, Farinpour, Sennett, Bowers, Legorreta, 2001). As with other chronic illnesses, SM skills are poorer among patients with limited reading skills (Williams, Baker, Honig, Lee, Nowlan, 1998).

While not claimed to be representative, one study of asthmatics presenting to an emergency room found that 62% were undertreated with medications when compared to the consensus guidelines and 87% did not have a written plan of action. During the asthma attack, 89% did not begin or increase use of an inhaled steroid; 31% thought short-acting brochodilator drugs were asthma preventers; 48% didn't own a peak flow (PF) meter (to detect deterioration in lung function); only 9% determined their peak expiratory flow daily, which means the others are likely to underestimate disease severity; and 40% smoked (Taylor, Auble, Calhoun, Mosesso, 1999). This latter proportion is higher than in the general population, of whom 22% to 25% smoke.

Almost 75% of admissions for asthma are avoidable, and potentially preventable factors are common in deaths from asthma. At least 40% of people with asthma do not react appropriately when their symptoms worsen, and more than half of patients admitted with acute asthma have had alarming symptoms for at least a week before admission. As many as 60% of asthmatic patients are poor at judging their dyspnea (Lahdensuo, 1999).

Because the course of the disease is highly variable, it is important for each patient to know his or her unique symptoms and triggers.

Standards for Self-Management Preparation

SM plans are advocated in most national guidelines on managing asthma, especially for persons with moderate to severe asthma and patients with a history of severe exacerbations. The purpose of these plans is to help patients self-manage their asthma at home through treatment adjustments in response to changes in symptoms or in peak expiratory flow rate. SM plans are especially important for patients with moderate to severe asthma and those with a history of severe exacerbations. Effective SM during a crisis is the desired goal (Radeos et al., 2001).

Data from focus groups (Jones, Pill, Adams, 2000) show that this guideline is infrequently implemented and that patients and health professionals are at best ambivalent about the potential usefulness of SM plans. In this study, general practitioners believed that patients didn't have the capacity for SM and that plans were difficult to achieve in everyday practice. Patients with mild to moderate asthma preferred to manage it as an intermittent acute disorder and were uncomfortable with a SM plan that reinforced the notion that asthma is a chronic, ongoing disease needing monitoring and managing.

Effective Interventions and Measurement Instruments

Asthma treatment is aimed at decreasing airway inflammation. Essential components of asthma education include the following: basic facts about asthma, role of quick-relief and long-term control medications, correct use of metered-dose inhalers and spacer use, self-monitoring, environmental control strategies to decrease exposure, and knowledge of rescue action for acute episodes. SM preparation goes beyond this preparation to develop the skills, judgment, and confidence needed to direct therapy within a framework set by health care providers but made the patient's own by his or her experience (sometimes called guided SM).

Figure 8.1 describes reasons for asthma SM skills to be developed, lists warning signs of asthma exacerbation, and identifies patients suitable for guided SM. Clear peak flow charts or pocket-sized cards with colors to mark different action limits can be used as indicated. Care required for severe asthma is complex and difficult — involving avoidance of multiple common environmental stimuli; taking several medications, each on different schedules with different side effects; and managing exacerbations (Lahdensuo, 1999).

A summary of 25 individual studies shows that SM preparation that involves self-monitoring by either expiratory flow or symptoms, coupled with regular medical review and a written action plan, appears to improve health outcomes for adults with asthma. Compared with usual care, SM preparation reduced hospitalizations, ED visits and unscheduled visits to the doctor, days off work, and nocturnal asthma. Measures of lung function were little changed, however.

Training programs that enable people to adjust their medication using a written action plan appear to be more effective than are other forms of asthma SM. Such a plan is individualized to the patient's underlying asthma severity and treatment and is produced for the purpose of patient SM of asthma exacerbations. It informs the patient about when and how to modify medications and to access the medical system in response to worsening asthma. Individualization of plans is developed from personal interviews and from SM during a baseline period (Gibson et al., 2002).

Widespread evidence of problems with delivery of care, limited knowledge, and poor asthma SM skills has been found among patients with severe asthma. There is also evidence that matters needn't be this way. With an inner-city minority

Asthma SM: Overview

Reasons for self-management of asthma

- Insidious deterioration (common in asthma)
- Three-quarters of asthma exacerbations resulting in hospital care are preventable
- Nearly half of patients react inappropriately to asthma exacerbations
- Poor perception of deteriorating dyspnea
- Proved value of patient education in the treatment of asthma
- Poor compliance (30% to 40%) with asthma drugs

Self-management skills

Patients should:

- Accept that asthma is a long-term and treatable disease
- Be able to accurately describe asthma and its treatment
- Actively participate in the control and management of their asthma
- Identify factors that make their asthma worse
- Be able to describe strategies for avoidance or reduction of exacerbating factors
- Recognize the signs and symptoms of worsening asthma
- Follow a prescribed written treatment plan
- Use correct technique for taking drugs including inhalants by metered-dose inhalers, dry-powder inhalers, diskhalers, spacers, or nebulizers
- Take appropriate action to prevent and treat symptoms in different situations
- Use medical resources appropriately for routine and acute care
- Monitor symptoms and objective measures of asthma control

- Identify barriers to compliance (adherence) to the treatment plan
- Address specific problems that have an impact on their individual condition

Warning signs of asthma exacerbation

- Increased dyspnea
- A combination of increased wheeze, cough, or mucus secretion
- Nocturnal asthma
- Increased use of short-acting sympathomimetics
- Increased exercise-induced asthma
- Decreased morning peak expiratory flow values

Patients suitable for guided self-management

Patients with:

- Moderate or severe asthma
- Variable disease
- History of emergency room visits owing to asthma
- Bad perception of the severity of the disease
- Good cooperation

Pocket card action guide

- Asthma under control: peak expiratory flow values greater than 85% of personal best — use regular treatment
- Asthma getting worse: peak expiratory flow values less than 85% of personal best — double dose of inhaled steroids
- Asthma severe: peak expiratory flow values less than 70% of personal best — start course of oral prednisone
- Asthma emergency: peak expiratory flow values less than 50% of personal best — go to emergency room immediately

Source: Lahdensuo, A. (1999). Guided self-management of asthma — how to do it. *British Medical Journal 319,* 759–760. Reprinted with permission from the BMJ Publishing Group.

FIGURE 8.1

population, George and colleagues (1999) were able to achieve significant decreases in ED visits and hospitalizations compared with a control group and significant cost savings to the managed care organization by using repetitive teaching sessions with clinical nurse specialists during hospitalization. Such inpatient programs are likely to reach patients who come in through the ED and are likely to be readmitted, thereby targeting patients who are high users of health care resources.

As with other chronic diseases, availability of SM preparation is of concern. Although action plans have been found to be effective, about half of patients in one study were not provided them by their physicians (Douglass et al., 2002). Most patients presenting to the ED with acute asthma do not have adequate primary care or exposure to SM preparation and so are at risk for poor asthma outcomes. Even so, a survey of 77 EDs participating in a multicenter trial found only 16% offering asthma SM preparation. No surveys of asthma SM preparation in community health care organizations or HMOs have been reported. This pattern of a lack of services reinforces patients' views that asthma is a series of acute events rather than a disease of chronic airway inflammation (Emond, Reed, Graff, Clark, Camargo, 2000).

Other studies (Harris, Shearer, 2001) show that preparation for SM is both an educational and a developmental process, with the desired end state being the ability to lead an unconstrained lifestyle. Patients who practice SM can readily articulate a detailed management plan for asthma control, including a range of signals of potential deterioration. To reach this end state, a long-term true partnership with a health provider seems essential to gaining sufficient skill and confidence. Many asthmatic patients acquire SM skills when they are asymptomatic; they are therefore deprived of the immediate opportunity to perform skills that actually control their asthma. Thus repeated assessment of individuals' performance is necessary to ensure that they can actually carry out their skills when they need them (Caplan, Creer, 2001).

Table 8.1 describes the attitudes, skills, and knowledge believed to be required for asthma SM (Partridge, Hill, 2000). To date, little evidence has been gathered about which methods,

TABLE 8.1 Attitudes, Skills, and Knowledge Required by a Patient with Asthma to Manage the Disease Effectively

- Acceptance that asthma is a long-term treatable disease
- The ability to describe accurately asthma and its treatment
- Active participation in the control and management of their asthma
- Identification of factors that make their asthma worse
- The ability to describe strategies for avoidance or reduction of exacerbating factors
- The ability to recognize the signs and symptoms of worsening asthma
- Following the prescribed treatment plan
- Correct administration of inhaled medications using an appropriate device (metered-dose inhaler, breath-actuated inhaler, spacer and nebulizer)
- Taking appropriate action to prevent and treat symptoms in different situations
- Using medical resources appropriately for routine and acute care
- Monitoring symptoms and objective measures of asthma control
- Identification of barriers to adherence to the treatment plan
- Addressing specific problems that have an impact on their condition

Source: Partridge, M. R., Hill, S. R. (2000). Enhancing care for people with asthma: The role of communication, education, training, and self-management. *European Respiratory Journal 16*, 333–348.

aids, content, and amount of interaction achieve the best results. Asthma SM preparation has been shown to increase SE and internality in health locus of control but it has not yet been shown that these changes mediate improvements in asthma SM. Active problem solving is effective. There is a dearth of interventions that address beliefs, behavior, and perceptions, even though it may be possible to train patients to improve their perceptions of airway obstruction. Attention to emotions is also important as panic and depression, which are particularly common in children, have direct psychophysiological effects on the lungs as well as affecting SM (Lehrer, Feldman, Giardino, Song, Schmaling, 2002; Partridge, Hill, 2002).

Follow-up for most asthma SM programs is a few months. Caplan and Creer (2001) followed patients six to seven years after their SM course and found that all continued to use these skills to some degree.

Asthma Self-Management in Children

Asthma affects nearly 5 million children younger than 18 years of age and is responsible for three times more school absences annually than any other cause. Children do no better with adherence to treatment guidelines than do adults. Of those who presented at an urban tertiary care children's hospital ED, 71% did not have a written action plan, 89% did not maintain a symptom diary, and 66% did not use their peak flow meters (Scarfone, Zorc, Capraro, 2001).

Families also seem to develop SM beliefs and capabilities in successive phases (Zimmerman, Bonner, Evans, Mellins, 1999). In the first phase of asthma symptom avoidance, periodic cough or wheezing is not perceived to be asthma. In the second phase, this perception gives way to acceptance but reactive response to acute episodes. Phase 3 is characterized by following doctor's orders but being unskilled and lacking confidence at preventing severe episodes. In phase 4, true self-regulation begins, including adjusting medication on the basis of signs and symptoms, in consultation with health professionals. In earlier phases, families are unresponsive to SM training. SM should be envisioned as a complex developmental process rather than as a single educational episode.

A number of validated pediatric asthma education programs exist; those developed and studied throughout the 1990s are described in Table 8.2. Further details about these programs and descriptions of others developed earlier may be found in Velsor-Friedrich and Srof (2000). The programs have demonstrated improvement on measures such as frequency of asthma attack and symptoms, medication adherence, and SM skills (Lehrer, Feldman, Giardino, Song, Schmaling, 2002). Overall, children who participated in these programs experienced fewer ED and unscheduled physician visits, improvement in physical

Name of Program	Sources	Goals of Program	Program Description	Target Audience	Critique
A+ Asthma Club Developed in 1991 by the Division of Children's Health Promotion, Department of Community and Family Medicine at the Georgetown University School of Medicine. Funding by NHLBI.	Schneider, S. L., Richard, M., Huss, K., Huss, R. W., Thompson, L. C., Butz, A. M., Eggleston, P. A., Kolodner, K. B., Rand, C. S., Malveaux, F. J. (1997). Moving health care education into the community. *Nursing Management*, 28(9), 40–43.	1. Fewer days of restricted activity 2. Appropriate management of acute episodes 3. Reduced emergency visits 4. Increased use of preventive medical care The A+ program is designed to promote the following activities: 1. Recognition and avoidance of asthma triggers 2. Recognition of clues to asthma attack 3. Correct use of medicines 4. Communication with parents, physician, and teacher about asthma management	A+ Asthma Club Content Outline Session 1: 1. What I know and want to know about asthma 2. What it's like when asthma is under control 3. What I want to be when I grow up Session 2: 1. Introduction to medicines 2. How to relax 3. What to do when attacks start, clues that an attack is starting Session 3: 1. Things that start asthma attacks 2. What to do in the room where I sleep 3. Other things I can do to keep asthma attacks from starting Session 4: 1. Problems with taking asthma medicines 2. Taking medicines the right way 3. How I remember to take them 4. Practicing with inhalers and spacers 5. Talking with doctors and nurses	African Americans grades 1–6 living in the inner city. School setting.	Presented in a sensitive, well-organized, and easy-to-follow format. A well-developed asthma education program for school-aged children.

(continued)

Name of Program	Sources	Goals of Program	Program Description	Target Audience	Critique
			Session 5: Making Choices about Asthma 1. Using STAR to make choices 2. Problems I have at school Session 6: Running, Playing, and Sports 1. How asthma medicines can help 2. How to talk to my parents about it 3. How to talk to my doctor about it (taken from p. 42 of Schneider article)		
Behavioral Self-Management Program	Colland, V. T. (1994). Learning to cope with asthma: A behavioural self-management program for children. *Patient Education and Counseling, 22,* 141–152.	The goal of the program is to improve skills in coping with asthma.	There are 10 one-hour sessions that use a combination of self-management training and cognitive behavioral therapy in a group, using games and learning materials specifically designed for the school-aged child. Program objectives include: 1. To increase the child's knowledge and understanding of asthma medicine and to practice correct inhalation technique 2. To positively influence the child's attitude toward accepting the illness and the need for medication 3. To increase self-efficacy concerning the child's management of asthma 4. To train the child in self-management activities	Children aged 8–13 years.	The multifaceted approach combines developmental and psychological theory, cognitive behavioral therapy, group therapy, and self-management training. Findings from a study using this program demonstrated highly significant differences in favor of the experimental group on both psychological and medical variables.

Childhood Asthma Project Supported with funding from NHBLI	Hendricson, W., Wood, P., Homberto, A., Hidalgo, A., Ramirez, A., Kromer, M., Selva, M., Parcel, G. (1996). Implementation of individualized patient education for Hispanic children with asthma. *Patient Education and Counseling, 29(2)*, 155–165. Hendricson, W. D., Wood, P. R., Hidalgo, H. A., Kromer, M. E., Parcel, G. S., Ramirez, A. G. (1994). Implementation of a physician education intervention. *Archives of Pediatric Adolescent Medicine, 148*, 595–601.	Increase the confidence in implementing national guidelines for asthma management To reduce morbidity among Hispanic children with asthma	The childhood asthma consists of two branches: 1. *A Pediatric Resident Educational Curriculum* with a clinic-based pediatric educational curriculum. The curriculum was designed with Hispanic patients as the primary focus. The program is based on *The Guidelines for the Diagnosis and Management of Asthma (GDMA)* developed by the Expert Panel of the National Asthma Education Program. Teaching strategies include focus groups, computer-based assessments of asthma knowledge, lectures, skill development seminars, mentoring with attending physicians, pocket cards and posters, access to peak flow and spirometry data, and interactive computer-based learning instruction. 2. *The Pediatric Education Component* consists of four phases: "baseline assessment, the educational intervention, application, and maintenance of learned behaviors" (Hendricson et al., 1995, p. 157) • Baseline assessment: Including learning goals, physical assessment, health beliefs and behaviors, and asthma knowledge. • Educational intervention: Including recognition of asthma symptoms, medication management, response to acute asthma symptoms, minimization of exposure to triggers, appropriate levels of physical	Medical residents and Hispanic children aged 6–16 years.	Closely linked with *Guidelines for the Diagnosis and Management of Asthma* developed by the Expert Panel of the National Asthma Education Program.

(continued)

◈ TABLE 8.2 (continued)

Name of Program	Sources	Goals of Program	Program Description	Target Audience	Critique
			activity, and communication with health care personnel. Teaching methods included return demonstration, videotape role modeling, and contracting. The educational intervention included 4 modules, covered over a 6-week period, with 45-minute programs each week. • Application: Self-management behaviors were practiced at home during this phase. The application phase evaluated the opinion of child and parent as to degree of self-management. • Maintenance of learned behaviors. This stage occurred at 6, 12, 18, and 24 months post-intervention. Clinic visits at these times focused on patient adherence to self-monitoring skills.		
Roaring Adventures of Puff Developed by Shawna L. McGhan, Education Coordinator, Alberta Asthma	McGhan, S., Wells, H. M., Befus, D. (1998). The "Roaring Adventures of Puff": A childhood asthma education program. *Journal of Pediatric Health*	1. Optimal self-regulation 2. Reduced asthma symptoms 3. Enhanced quality of life 4. Decreased school absenteeism 5. Decreased health care use	"Six 60-minute sessions with interactive teaching strategies such as puppetry, games, role play, model building, and asthma diary interpretation" (pp. 192–193). Children establish their own goals and keep an action plan diary logging "symptoms, peak flow readings, medications, exposure to triggers, and physical activity" (p. 193). The program includes role	Children aged 7–12 and their families. To be used in the school setting.	Based on the well-recognized social cognitive theory by Bandura. Consistent with Canadian Consensus Guidelines on Asthma Management.

Centre University of Alberta	*Care, 12*(4), 191–195.	6. Self-efficacy 7. Increased internal motivation 8. Positive attitude	play in a way that assists children to make judgments and take appropriate response actions. The program also includes peer group support opportunities, games, and puppetry. The program includes the school personnel, child, and parents in developing the action plan.		
Wee Wheezers	Wilson, S. R., Scamagas, P., Grado, J., Norgaard, L., Starr, N. J., Eaton, S., Pomaville, K. (1998). The Fresno asthma project: A model intervention to control asthma in multiethnic, low-income, inner-city communities. *Health Education and Behavior, 25*(1), 79–98. Wilson, S. R., Latini, D., Starr, N., Loes, L., Page, A., Kubit, P. (1996).	1. To meet the educational needs of parents of children under the age of 7 years 2. To improve children's symptoms, parent's knowledge, attitudes, and asthma management practices	The program consists of four sessions. Two sessions are for parents alone, and two sessions are for parents and children. Parent sessions include instruction on the effects of asthma on the lungs, asthma medications, and trigger avoidance; videotapes that reinforce content are used. Children are taught to use metered-dose inhalers with spacers, recognize early warning signs and triggers, and seek help from parents/teachers.	Children aged 4–7 years and their parents.	One of the few programs for the younger child. Program includes an individually tailored written asthma action plan for use with routine medications and at-home management of acute episodes.

(continued)

159

◈ TABLE 8.2 (continued)

Name of Program	Sources	Goals of Program	Program Description	Target Audience	Critique
	Education of parents of infants and very young children with asthma. *Journal of Asthma, 33*(4), 239–254.				
You Can Control Asthma (YCCA)	Taggert, V. S., Zuckerman, A. E., Sly, M., Steinmueller, C., Newman, G., O'Brien, R. W., Schneider, S., Bellanti, J. A. (1991). You can control asthma: Evaluation of an asthma education program for hospitalized inner-city children. *Patient Education and Counseling, 17*(1), 35–47.	1. Increase patient and parent confidence 2. Increase patient and parent knowledge 3. Increase continuity of care	Three components: 1. Written materials: asthma control, asthma facts, asthma medications, referral phone numbers 2. Videotape presentations: asthma self-management 3. Interpersonal communication-discussions with health professionals	Hospitalized inner-city children aged 6–12 and their parents.	Due to the frequent absence of parents in the hospital setting, teaching directed toward parents is not highly emphasized. The program was originally developed for use in the emergency room setting and modified for inpatient use.

Source: Velsor-Friedrich, B., Srof, B. (2000). Asthma self-management programs for children. Part I: Description of the programs. *Journal of Child and Family Nursing 3*(2), 85–97.

and social activities, better asthma SM and enhanced SE, fewer school absences, and improved school performance (Velsor-Friedrich, Srof, 2000).

Other innovative programs have been developed or used with new groups. Using an interactive educational computer program of a child going through simulated daily events, Asthma Control taught SM to children ages 3 to 12 (Homer et al., 2000). A similar program, Health Buddy, which was designed for inner-city children, showed good outcomes, including being less likely to report limitation in activities and better peak flow readings in comparison with the control group (Guendelman, Meade, Benson, Chen, Samuels, 2002). A structured peer-led program for adolescents known as Triple A (Adolescent Asthma Action) to promote SM also showed improved quality of life and significant decreases in school absenteeism in the intervention group relative to the control group. Asthma attacks at school increased in the control group only (Shah et al., 2001). Students learned how to educate their peers about asthma and its management by using games, videos, worksheets, and discussions.

ASTHMA SE SCALE

This instrument (Mancuso, Rincon, McCulloch, Charlson, 2001) (Figure 8.2) asks patients to rate their confidence in avoiding an asthma attack in 80 different situations, encompassing activities, interactions with others, and emotions. An overall mean score is calculated by summing items from 1 (no confidence) to 5 (very confident). SE was one of the strongest predictors of quality-of-life outcomes. In contrast with SM in other chronic diseases, SE is rarely addressed in asthma.

An additional evaluation tool is checklists for correct use of instruments, as shown in Figure 8.3. Aerosol drugs — both bronchodilators and steriods — remain a mainstay of asthma treatment. Metered-dose inhalers (MDI) are convenient and portable, but a significant proportion of patients do not know how to use them correctly (i.e., coordinating timing of the cannister activation with inhalation). Some patients cannot learn

The Asthma Self-Efficacy Scale

The following items describe situations in which asthma attacks may occur. Read each description, and as vividly as possible try to imagine yourself in that situation. Then assess how confident you are that you could successfully avoid or manage an asthma attack if one occurred. If you are absolutely certain that you could successfully cope with that situation, mark "e" in the accompanying box. If you have no confidence in your ability to successfully cope with a given situation, mark "a." It is possible your confidence may vary from situation to situation.

a) No confidence   **b)** Little confidence   **c)** Somewhat confident   **d)** Pretty confident   **e)** Very confident

How confident are you that you would be able to avoid an asthma attack in these situations?

1. When I become too tired. ☐
2. When I face into the wind. ☐
3. When I eat some types of foods (especially spicy foods). ☐
4. When I face the air conditioning. ☐
5. When I go into cold weather from a warm place (e.g., a warm house or car). ☐
6. When I experience emotional stress or become upset. ☐
7. When I am around dust. ☐
8. When I am around strong smells or fumes (e.g., paints, varnishes, perfumes, soaps, sprays, etc.). ☐
9. When I take some types of medication (including aspirin). ☐
10. When I go upstairs too fast. ☐
11. When I am around cigarette smoke. ☐
12. When I hurry or rush around. ☐
13. When I exercise or physically exert myself. ☐
14. When there is a sudden change in temperature (hot or cold). ☐
15. When I experience sudden excitement. ☐
16. When I lift heavy objects. ☐
17. When there is humidity in the air. ☐

18. When I yell at the kids. ☐
19. When I am around animals. ☐
20. When I am lying prone in bed. ☐
21. When it rains. ☐
22. During very hot weather. ☐
23. When I experience stress or anger. ☐
24. When there is pollen in the air. ☐
25. When I go into a musty, damp room. ☐
26. When I laugh excessively. ☐
27. When I am in a hot, dry house in the wintertime. ☐
28. When I talk to people who are angry or upset. ☐
29. When I am trying to meet a deadline. ☐
30. When I mow grass or am around freshly mowed grass. ☐
31. After I eat. ☐
32. When I am in a close, confined space (e.g., a car or small room). ☐
33. When I wear scratchy material (e.g., wool). ☐
34. When I go out into the damp air. ☐
35. When I use nasal sprays. ☐

FIGURE 8.2

36. When I am around mold. ☐
37. When I am around a fireplace or woodburning stove. ☐
38. When I use an electric blanket. ☐
39. When I am around certain kinds of carpeting. ☐
40. When I sleep on a feather pillow. ☐
41. When I use detergents with fabric softeners. ☐
42. When I am in woods or fields. ☐
43. When I vacuum. ☐
44. When I drink certain kinds of alcoholic beverages. ☐
45. When I get an infection (throat, sinus, colds, the flu). ☐
46. When I use some types of makeup. ☐
47. When I dance. ☐
48. When I am at the doctor's office and experience tension or anxiety. ☐
49. When I am around pollution. ☐
50. When I smell chlorine fumes at pools. ☐
51. When I am in a closed space with flowers. ☐
52. When I wear winter clothing and become overheated. ☐
53. When I overeat. ☐
54. When I take a hot shower. ☐
55. When I have a full bladder. ☐
56. When I am pregnant. ☐
57. When I cry. ☐

58. When I am around people. ☐
59. A few days before menstruation begins. ☐
60. When I breathe improperly. ☐
61. When I don't drink enough fluids. ☐
62. When my diet is not properly balanced. ☐
63. When I am afraid. ☐
64. When I experience the loss of a valued object. ☐
65. When I am anxious. ☐
66. When I swim in an outdoor pool. ☐
67. When there are problems in my family. ☐
68. When I am around bath powders. ☐
69. When I am near a field that is being plowed. ☐
70. When I go into a hot place after coming in from the cold. ☐
71. When I come home from a trip. ☐
72. When I am around plants. ☐
73. When the weather is simultaneously hot and humid. ☐
74. When I am angry. ☐
75. When I get a skin allergy. ☐
76. When my sinuses are draining. ☐
77. When I am around hay. ☐
78. During harvest time. ☐
79. When I am around a kerosene heater. ☐
80. When I exercise in a room that is not adequately ventilated. ☐

Source: Tobin, D. L., Wigal, J., Winder, J. A., Holroyd, K. A., Creer, T. L. (1987). The Asthma Self-Efficacy Scale, *Annals of Allergy* 59, 273–277.

FIGURE 8.2 *(continued)*

Checklists for Proper Inhalation Techniques

Checklist for proper inhalation technique of MDI	Checklist for proper inhalation technique of BAI
___(a) Takes off cap	___(a) Takes off cap
___(b) Shakes	___(b) Shakes
___(c) Holds inhaler upright	___(c) Holds inhaler upright
___(d) Activates inhaler during inspiration	___(d) Lifts lever each time
___(e) Inhales slowly and deeply	___(e) Closes mouth around inhaler
___(f) Holds breath for 5–10 seconds	___(f) Inhales slowly and deeply after the medication is triggered
___(g) One puff at a time	___(g) Holds breath for 5–10 seconds
___(h) 15–60 seconds between puffs	___(h) One puff at a time
	___(i) 15–60 seconds between puffs

MDI = Metered-dose inhaler   BAI = Breath-activated inhaler

Source: Rydman, R. J., Sonenthal, K., Tadimeti, L., Butki, N., McDermott, M. F. (1999). Evaluating the outcome of two teaching methods of breath-activated inhaler in an inner city asthma clinic. *Journal of Medical Systems 23,* 349–356. Reprinted with permission from Kluwer Academic/Plenum Publishers.

FIGURE 8.3

the technique despite repeated instructions, although spacer devices help. The breath-activated inhaler (BAI) has been developed as an adjunctive therapy to help promote proper techniques. In an inner-city asthma population, patients could retain proper knowledge of BAI with written instructions. In general, however, patients need continuous reinforcement as well to use inhalers correctly (Rydman, Sonenthal, Tadimeti, Butki, McDermott, 1999).

Action Plan Decisions (Figure 8.4) includes scenarios that might be faced by an asthmatic child. Participants in a SM preparation were asked to suggest a solution to each scenario, followed by discussion of them (Child Asthma Management Program Research Group, 1998).

Additional instruments relevant to SM may be found in Redman (2003).

A number of questions remain. Studies of the cost-effectiveness of asthma SM preparation have found variable results. The most

---

Action Plan Decisions

- You are visiting the zoo with a friend. Your eyes begin to water and your chin itches. What should you do?

- You go to a ball game with your friend and someone next to you starts smoking. Pretty soon your chest starts to feel tight. What should you do?

- Your friends want you to rollerblade. After about ten minutes you start to cough and can't catch your breath. What should you do?

- After gym class your chest feels tight and you measure your peak flow number. Your number is in the red zone and you use your rescue inhaler. Five minutes later you use your peak flow meter again and you are still in the red zone. What should you do?

- You have a cold and your peak flow number keeps dropping into the yellow zone. For the last day you have been taking your rescue inhaler every four hours. What should you do?

★ Congratulations! You made ____ terrific decisions!

Source: Childhood Asthma Management Program Research Group. (1998). Design and implementation of a patient education center for the childhood asthma management program. *Annals of Allergy, Asthma, Immunology 81,* 571–581. Used with permission.

FIGURE 8.4

favorable show an $11.22 benefit for every $1 spent (Lahdensuo, 1999; Lehrer, Feldman, Giardino, Song, Schmaling, 2002). The long-term influence of self-treatment on the course of asthma remains unknown. Also, which patients might profit most from SM programs is also unknown.

Canada has established a National Asthma Educator Certification program, and Quebec has a well-organized and cooperating system of asthma SM preparation centers. To ensure referral of those most in need of education, patients treated for asthma in EDs or those noted by pharmacists to be using excessive amounts of bronchodilator therapy are now referred directly to Asthma Education Centers (Cowie, Cicutto, Boulet, 2001).

◈ COPD Self-Management Preparation

There has been an increase in morbidity and mortality due to chronic obstructive pulmonary disease (COPD) in the Western world over the last few decades. Despite this trend, virtually no literature on SM preparation for this group is available. A cluster of studies done by a Norwegian group seems modeled after asthma SM preparation with an individual treatment plan. This work is not, however, based on theoretical models characteristic of SM (SE, problem solving, belief models, stages of change) and uses goals and teaching techniques more characteristic of patient education (information giving, demonstration, persuasion) than of SM preparation. Experimental interventions did show cost savings, including decreased physician visits and amounts of short-acting rescue medications, over control groups (Gallefos, Bakke, 1999, 2000, 2002).

References

Caplin, D. L., Creer, T. L. (2001). A self-management program for adult asthma. III. Maintenance and relapse of skills. *Journal of Asthma 38,* 343–356.

Childhood Asthma Management Program Research Group. (1998). Design and implementation of a patient education center for the childhood asthma management program. *Annals of Allergy, Asthma, Immunology 81,* 571–581.

Cowie, R. L., Cicutto, L., Boulet, L. (2001). Asthma education and management programs in Canada. *Canadian Respiratory Journal 8,* 416–420.

Douglass, J., et al. (2002). A qualitative study of action plans for asthma. *British Medical Journal 324,* 1003–1005.

Emond, S. D., Reed, C. R., Graff, L. G., Clark, S., Camargo, C. A. (2000). Asthma education in the emergency department. *Annals of Emergency Medicine 36,* 204–211.

Gallefoss, F., Bakke, P. S. (2002). Cost-benefit and cost-effectiveness analysis of self-management in patients with COPD — a one-year follow-up randomized, controlled trial. *Respiratory Medicine 96,* 424–431.

Gallefoss, F., Bakke, P. S. (2000). Impact of patient education and self-management on morbidity in asthmatics and patients with chronic obstructive pulmonary disease. *Respiratory Medicine 94,* 279–287.

Gallefos, F., Bakke, P. S. (1999). How does patient education and self-management among asthmatics and patients with chronic obstructive pulmonary disease affect medication? *American Journal of Respiratory and Critical Care Medicine 160*, 2000–2005.

George, M. R., et al. (1999). A comprehensive educational program improves clinical outcome measures in inner-city patients with asthma. *Archives of Internal Medicine 159*, 1710–1715.

Gibson, P. G., et al. (2002). *Self-management education and regular practitioner review for adults with asthma (Cochrane Review)*. In The Cochrane Library, Issue 2. Oxford: Update Software.

Guendelman, S., Meade, K., Benson, M., Chen, Y. Q., Samuels, S. (2002). Improving asthma outcomes and self-management behaviors of inner-city children. *Archives of Pediatric and Adolescent Medicine 156*, 114–120.

Harris, G. S., Shearer, A. G. (2001). Beliefs that support the behavior of people with asthma: A qualitative investigation. *Journal of Asthma 38*, 427–434.

Homer, C., et al. (2000). An evaluation of an innovative multimedia educational software program for asthma management: Report of a randomized, controlled trial. *Pediatrics 106*, 210–215.

Jones, A., Pill, R., Adams, S. (2000). Qualitative study of views of health professionals and patients on guided self management plans for asthma. *British Medical Journal 321*, 1507–1510.

Lahdensuo, A. (1999). Guided self management of asthma — how to do it. *British Medical Journal 319*, 759–760.

Lehrer, P., Feldman, J., Giardino, N., Song, H., Schmaling, K. (2002). Psychological aspects of asthma. *Journal of Consulting and Clinical Psychology 70*, 691–711.

Liu, X., Farinpour, R., Sennett, C., Bowers, B. W., Legorreta, A. P. (2001). Improving the quality of care of patients with asthma: The example of patients with severely symptomatic disease. *Journal of Evaluation in Clinical Practice 7*, 261–269.

Mancuso, C. A., Rincon, M., McCulloch, C. E., Charlson, M. E. (2001). Self-efficacy, depressive symptoms and patients' expectations predict outcomes in asthma. *Medical Care 39*, 1326–1338.

Partridge, M. R., Hill, S. R. (2000). Enhancing care for people with asthma: The role of communication, education, training and self-management. *European Respiratory Journal 16*, 333–348.

Radeos, M. S., et al. (2001). Risk factors for lack of asthma self-management knowledge among ED patients not on inhaled steroids. *American Journal of Surgery Medicine 19,* 253–259.

Redman, B. K. (2003). *Measurement tools in patient education,* 2nd ed. New York: Springer Publishing.

Reinke, L. F., Hoffman, L. (2000). Asthma education: Creating a partnership. *Heart & Lung 29,* 225–236.

Rydman, R. J., Sonenthal, K., Tadimeti, L., Butki, N., McDermott, M. F. (1999). Evaluating the outcome of two teaching methods of breath-activated inhaler in an inner city asthma clinic. *Journal of Medical Systems 23,* 349–356.

Scarfone, R. J., Zorc, J. J., Capraro, G. A. (2001). Patient self-management of acute asthma: Adherence to national guidelines a decade later. *Pediatrics 108,* 1332–1338.

Shah, S., et al. (2001). Effect of peer led programme for asthma education in adolescents: Cluster randomized controlled trial. *British Medical Journal 322,* 583–585.

Taylor, D. M., Auble, T. E., Calhoun, W. J., Mosesso, V. N. (1999). Current outpatient management of asthma shows poor compliance with international consensus guidelines. *Chest 116,* 1638–1645.

Velsor-Friedrich, B., Srof, B. (2000). Asthma self-management programs for children. Part I: Description of the programs. *Journal of Child and Family Nursing 3,* 85–97.

Williams, M. V., Baker, D. W., Honig, E. G., Lee, T. M., Nowlan, A. (1998). Inadequate literacy is a barrier to asthma knowledge and self-care. *Chest 114,* 1008–1015.

Zimmerman, B. J., Bonner, S., Evans, D., Mellins, R. B. (1999). Self-regulating childhood asthma: A developmental model of family change. *Health Education & Behavior 26,* 55–71.

9

Diabetes Self-Management Preparation

 pproximately 16 million people in the United States have diabetes, two-thirds of whom have been diagnosed. Diabetes patients account for nearly 6% of the total population and 11% of those aged 65 and older. Diabetes is the seventh leading cause of death, with mortality coming primarily from heart disease, and it accounts for 40% of all new end-stage renal disease cases. Ninety percent of patients have type 2 diabetes, which is strongly associated with obesity and age but is also increasing in overweight children and adolescents. Fewer than 10% of patients are able to control type 2 diabetes through diet and exercise alone, and there is a growing tendency to use insulin to achieve tighter blood glucose control in this population (Gonder-Frederick, Cox, Ritterband, 2002).

Diabetes care without adequate SM preparation can be regarded as substandard and unethical care. Surveys of managed care organizations have documented that substandard care is the norm for people with diabetes who do not use insulin. It is unusual to have formal programs after the basic diabetes education. Arguably, the tradition of diabetes education and acknowledgment of its importance by national organizations and, to some degree, by reimbursement policy puts it in a more favorable position than does SM preparation for other chronic diseases. One study (Yawn, Zyzanski, Goodwin, Gotler, Stange, 2001) found that compared with patients with other chronic diseases, visits to family physicians by persons with diabetes were longer and devoted a greater proportion of time to nutrition counseling, health education and feedback on results, negotiation, and assessment of compliance.

Large trials [such as the Diabetes Control and Complications Trial (DCCT) and the United Kingdom Prospective Diabetes Study] have demonstrated that tight glycemic control can improve microvascular outcomes. These findings meant that overnight, large numbers of patients were expected to follow a demanding, intensive treatment regimen that was previously recommended only for those most highly motivated in SM and yielded increased risk for episodes of severe hypoglycemia. Hypertension and hyperlipidemia must also be controlled. In gestational diabetes, mothers must quickly learn and adapt to a demanding treatment regimen to avoid fetal complications, typically in the third trimester (Gonder-Frederick, Cox, Ritterband, 2002).

Instead of a specific diabetic diet, authorities now recommend a healthy low-fat meal plan individually tailored to patient lifestyle, culture, and ethnicity, Nevertheless, food still must be monitored closely and patients typically quantify their intake by some method.

In the adolescent and young adult female population, eating disorders are far more prevalent as individuals manipulate insulin dose to control weight. Anxiety disorders appear to be more prevalent in people with diabetes and are associated with poor metabolic control. Those with high trait anxiety misattribute bodily symptoms to hypoglycemia, which can lead to unnecessary treatment. Clinical depression occurs in 15% to 20% of patients and interferes with adequate self-treatment; diabetes is a significant risk factor for development of psychiatric problems for all age groups.

Peer relationships have important influence on diabetes SM, especially in adolescents, but have not received important empirical attention. It is also understood that adolescents commonly lack the cognitive ability to manipulate the multiple factors inherent in diabetes SM (Schilling, Grey, Knafl, 2002). Children are dependent on their families; those who show less conflict and more cohesion experience fewer episodes of ketoacidosis and severe hypoglycemia and less deterioration in metabolic control. Episodes of severe hypoglycemia can have a detrimental effect on cognitive-motor abilities, especially in the developing brain, and achieving tight control in young children is difficult. Even mild hypoglycemia can cause performance deficits on a variety of tasks, with many subjects remaining unaware of their shortfalls (Gonder-Frederick, Cox, Ritterband, 2002).

Personal health beliefs and models of illness and SE predict SM across a wide range of behaviors. Hampson, Glasgow, and Strycker (2000) found patients' personal models (representations of illness) were stronger and more consistent predictors of outcome (eating patterns, physical functioning, glycosylated hemoglobin) than was depression. For diabetes, the components of adult and adolescent personal models have been identified, replicated, and demonstrated to be associated with SM outcomes both concurrently and prospectively. Patients' beliefs concerning the seriousness of their diabetes and their beliefs about effectiveness of their treatment are most predictive.

Psychosocial problems frequently emerge in youths several years post-diagnosis. Adults frequently have diabetes burnout, although few longitudinal studies of psychosocial adaptation to diabetes have been completed for any group.

There have been efforts to make the regimen more user-friendly. Functional insulin treatment (FIT; Howorka et al., 2000) allows patients free choice of food intake because they learn to dose their insulin according to their blood glucose levels and food intake either with multiple daily injections or a continuous pump. The opportunity to eat when and whatever the patient wants to eat (no meal planning) or even not to eat (fasting was made possible) can be expected to influence the perception of SE.

Standards for Self-Management Preparation

The American Diabetes Association standards evaluate the process and structure of the educational program: the organizational structure, mission, and goals; target population; educational needs and resources; involvement of professional staff and other stakeholders; coordinator with adequate experience; educational team that has regular continuing education; written curriculum with criteria for learning outcomes; development of educational plan for each participant; continuous quality improvement (Mensing et al., 2000).

Because outcomes for patients are poorly defined, metabolic measurement such as HbA1C, body mass index, and lipid levels are not infrequently used for monitoring outcomes of diabetes education. Although these outcomes may be affected indirectly by education, they are also influenced by factors such as medical management, making it difficult to describe the actual results of the educational intervention. It becomes crucial to identify unique outcome measures that can be specifically and consistently linked to the educational process (Peeples, Mulcahy, Tomky, Weaver, 2001).

Healthy People 2010 (U.S. Department of Health and Human Services, 2000) recommends diabetes SM preparation as a cornerstone of treatment for all people with diabetes, with a goal of increasing the 1998 baseline of the number of people who receive formal diabetes education from 40% to 60%. Goals of SM preparation are to optimize metabolic control and quality of life and to prevent acute and chronic complications while keeping costs acceptable. Fifty to eighty percent of people with diabetes have significant knowledge and skill deficits, and less than half of all people with type 2 diabetes achieve ideal glycemic control. The American Diabetes Association recommends assessing SM skills and knowledge at least annually and giving continuing education (Norris et al., 2002).

In addition, it is important to note that no recognized standards of care for the inpatient management of diabetes SM preparation exist. The overwhelming majority of hospitalizations for persons with diabetes occur for treatment of comorbidities such as cardiac conditions. Yet, diabetes management is rarely the focus of care, and glucose control and other diabetes-related care processes, including SM instruction before discharge, are inadequately addressed. In one study, 40% of the patients so admitted had important diabetes knowledge deficits. Development of a clinical path for type 2 diabetes as a secondary diagnosis and making glucose values prominent were associated with decreased frequency of prolonged and severe hyperglycemia and nosocomial infections. In the tertiary care medical center where the study was carried out, more than 10% of hospitalized patients had diagnostic codes for diabetes and on any given day 25% to 40% of these patients on the medical and surgical cardiac care units had diabetes (Roman, Chassin, 2001). Dialysis units are also regularly attended by large numbers of diabetes patients and hence represent additional sites for SM preparation (McMurray, Johnson, Davis, McDougall, 2002).

Effective Interventions and Measurement Instruments

A number of elements have been found useful in SM preparation (Glasgow et al., 2002):

- Assessment of current SM, beliefs, and barriers
- Collaborative goal setting
- Problem-solving and coping skills training to enhance patient SE
- Strategies to overcome barriers
- Individualized written action plans
- An iterative and self-correcting process rather than one-time activity
- Incorporating SM preparation as an integral part of the overall health care system rather than as a stand-alone, isolated activity

Many patients have received no assistance with SM. As many as half leave an office visit not knowing what they're supposed to do to care for themselves. An average of less than 1 minute of a 20-minute physician visit is spent giving patients any kind of information (Heisler, Reynard, Hayward, Smith, Kerr, 2002). Educated patients believe that the manual skills are relatively easy to acquire, whereas the skills required to solve problems and make decisions such as adaptation of doses of insulin are much more difficult (Bonnet, Gagnayre, d'Ivernois, 2001).

Learning SM involves not only skill and problem solving but also phases of integration of the approach to diabetes. A group of expert self-managers of long-term type 1 diabetes had moved through some or all of the following phases:

1. Passive compliance, in which they craved structure and rules
2. Naive experimentation, in which they altered insulin or diet but lacked the skills to do so effectively
3. Rebellion, in which they ignored the diet or alcohol restrictions, hiding their need for insulin or falsifying or neglecting glucometer readings
4. Active control, in which they paid attention to their bodies and subtle signs and made a conscious decision to assume control

They finally developed sufficient confidence, competence, and social support to assume active control in both familiar and unfamiliar SM situations.

The phases were not always distinct and at times overlapped. Some retained aspects of a previous phase until behaviors associated with the new phase were well integrated. Many shopped around for and demanded health professionals who acknowledged their expertise and agreed to collaborate in decisions, although most were unable to find such providers (Paterson, Thorne, 2000a).

On the other hand, many patients face significant barriers to learning. In the United States, 80% of patients with type 2 diabetes have completed only high school or less, compared with 40% of the general population. In one study (Schillinger et al., 2002), two-thirds of patients with a high school education or less had inadequate or marginal health literacy (a constellation of skills including the ability to perform the basic reading and numerical tasks required to function in the health care environment).

Inadequate health literacy is independently associated with worse glycemic control and higher rates of retinopathy. Standard diabetes education did not eliminate health literacy-related disparities in diabetes outcomes. These patients have lower levels of diabetes-related knowledge and are less likely to correctly interpret or act on SM results even after exposure to health education.

For example, only half of patients with inadequate literacy knew that feeling shaky, sweaty, and hungry meant one's blood sugar level was low, compared with 94% of patients with adequate functional health literacy. Only 38% of low-literacy patients knew the proper treatment for such symptoms, compared with 73% of literate patients. These scores occurred despite the fact that patients with inadequate literacy had attended formal educational classes. Measures of outcome were not significantly associated with literacy, however (Williams, Baker, Parker, Nurss, 1998).

Cognitive dysfunction is relatively common in elderly diabetics; Sinclair, Girling, and Bayer (2000) recommend routine screening of cognition in these individuals. Approximately one-fourth of the millions of Americans with type 2 diabetes experience depression. At some point on the continuum, these patients will display poorer SM ability.

Norris has provided a series of reports on the effectiveness of SM preparation, including a meta-analysis. This evidence shows that, on average, an intervention decreases glycosylated hemoglobin by 0.76% more than control at immediate follow-up, and by 0.26% at one to three months and at more than four months. For every 23.6 additional hours of contact between participant and educator, glycosylated hemoglobin decreases an additional 1%. Time of contact was found to be the only significant predictor in the meta-analysis; educational focus, group versus individual, timeframe, and person who delivered the education made no difference (Norris, Lau, Smith, Schmid, Engelgau, 2002).

In type 2 diabetes, 72 studies with short-term follow-up have shown positive effects of SM training on knowledge and accuracy of self-monitoring blood glucose (SMBG), self-reported dietary habits, and glycemic control. Effects of intervention on lipids, physical activity, weight, and blood pressure were variable. A variety of measurement instruments were used to test knowledge but frequently lacked documented reliability and validity. Most studies compare a more intensive intervention to basic care and education, as it is generally considered unethical to randomize a group to receive no education, thus minimizing the effects of the intervention. There is also frequently an inadequate description of the study interventions and participants, including representiveness of study populations. Data are insufficient to determine which behavioral tools and therapies are most advantageous (Norris, Engelgau, Narayan, 2001).

There is sufficient evidence to show that SM preparation is effective in community gathering places for adults with type 2 diabetes and in the home for adolescents with type 1 diabetes. Conversely, evidence is insufficient to assess effectiveness of SM interventions at work sites, at summer camps, in the home for type 2 diabetes patients, or for educating co-workers and school personnel about diabetes.

To date, there has been a strong emphasis on SMBG as a SM tool. Experts believe that it may provide important feedback for patients and providers, but little evidence indicates that it contributes to glycemic control in type 2 patients. Patients may have difficulty obtaining accurate measurements or be unable to respond to the results effectively, formal structural skills training can, however, improve type 1 patients' ability to perceive periods of glucose dysregulation. Type 1 patients may be unable to make appropriate adjustments before cognitive symptoms develop (Piette, Glasgow, 2001).

Cox, Gonder-Frederick, Kovatchev, and Clarke (2001) note there is a narrow window between a patient's detection of hypoglycemic symptoms and the need to self-treat while driving, and neuroglycemia, which impairs self-treatment. Trembling, uncoordination, and visual difficulties are symptoms. SM in this situation requires pulling off the road immediately to consume fast-acting carbohydrates and not resuming driving until both blood glucose and cognitive and motor functions recover. Only one-third of patients tested on a driving simulator managed this self-treatment. Behaviors required to achieve glycemic control are complex, are uniquely tailored to the individual, and cannot easily be captured in textbook-derived recommendations by practitioners (Paterson, Thorne, 2000b).

Foot care SM preparation is effective and can decrease the incidence of foot problems. For people whom a screening program finds to be at high risk for foot ulcer development, continuing and well-structured education supported by podiatry should be applied. One such program consisted of four two-hour sessions held over a week, providing SM skills about shoes and socks, walking barefoot, foot hygiene, callus care, nail cutting, water temperature checks, use of foot warming devices, bathroom surgery, use of foot care products, and methods of foot and shoe inspection. Seventy percent of patients complied with this program and changed inappropriate foot care behavior with an 8- to 22-fold decrease in foot ulceration; the study did not include a control group (Piette and Glasgow, 2001; Calle-Pascual et al., 2002).

Management of psychosocial problems is also important because they are a stronger predictor of mortality in diabetes patients than are many clinical and physiological variables. Depression — more common in patients with diabetes (15%) than in the general population — is associated with worse glycemic control, more health complications, and decreased quality of life. Anxiety disorders are common in adults with diabetes and are linked with poor glycemic control, and eating disorders are especially common in women with type 1 diabetes (Delamater et al., 2001). Some of these psychosocial issues can be at least partly self-managed, and many may affect the patient's ability to learn broader SM skills. Developmentally precipitated shifts in autonomy (which is essential to SM) also need to be managed so that they will strengthen skills in responsible independence.

Instruction has successfully been offered through automated telephone assessment and self-care educational calls with nurse follow-up. Automated calling systems use computer technology to deliver messages and collect information from patients using a touch-tone keypad or voice-response technology. For example, on the automated calls, patients can report barriers to SM and receive education and advice. This system allows the nurse to focus on those patients most in need of assistance. It can be language appropriate and has been used successfully with low-income patients (Piette and others, 2000). Also successful is an

Internet-based Diabetes Network (McKay, King, Eakin, Seeley, Glasgow, 2001).

It is possible to build into such interventions support from a personal coach as well as goal setting and weekly activities. Expansion of these methods is essential because SM preparation programs reach only a minority of those persons in need of them. Fewer than half of type 2 patients and fewer than 60% of type 1 patients have ever received diabetes education. Fiel, Glasgow, Boles, and McKay (2000) found that computer novices recruited from primary care physician practices did well with one Internet-based diabetes SM support program.

Development of a sustained partnership between patient and provider is also known to be associated with such favorable outcomes as fewer and shorter hospitalizations and ED visits, higher patient satisfaction, and increased likelihood of having problems identified by the provider (Parchman, Pugh, Noel, Larme, 2002).

Several other practices are important. All persons with diabetes should receive an assessment to determine their current SM educational needs annually and whenever lifestyle or treatment changes or signs of management problems or complications arise. New delivery patterns, such as use of ongoing chronic disease mini-clinics to address clinical, SM, and psychosocial needs, may allow for this kind of continuous service. Finally, combinations of postgraduate education for health professionals, patient education, and use of a nurse for follow-up were found in several studies to lead to improvements in patient outcomes as well as in the process of care (Renders et al., 2001).

Diabetes occurs disproportionately in minority populations. For example, Mexican Americans tend to be diagnosed at younger ages with more severe forms of diabetes complications. Culturally competent diabetes SM preparation has been prepared and tested with Mexican Americans with type 2 diabetes. Fifty-two contact hours were provided over 12 months by bilingual Mexican American nurses, dietitians, and community workers during three months of weekly instructional sessions in nutrition, SMBG, and exercise and six months of biweekly support group sessions to promote behavior change (see Table 9.1

◈ TABLE 9.1　Characteristics of the Intervention

Baseline	Intervention		Postintervention at 3, 6, and 12 Months
Measures	**Weekly Education Sessions (12 Weekly Meetings)**	**Support Group Sessions (14 Biweekly Meetings)**	
• Demographics (age, gender, age of diabetes diagnosis, etc.) • Acculturation • Family, medical, and medication history • Diabetes knowledge • Diabetes-related health beliefs • Glycosylated hemoglobin • Fasting blood glucose • Systolic and diastolic blood pressure • Total cholesterol: 　HDL cholesterol 　LDL cholesterol • Triglycerides	• Introduction • What is hyperglycemia? • Glucose self-monitoring • Dietary principles for Mexican American foods • Food preparation • Food labels (trip to grocery store) • Medications • Exercise • Hygiene: Illness days, foot care, etc. • Short-term complications: hyper- and hypoglycemia • Long-term complications • Family support and community resources	Format for each session is: • Review of previously learned content • Assessment of participants' knowledge and skills regarding area under discussion • Discussion of ongoing barriers to adopting healthy lifestyle changes—group problem solving • Demonstration of healthy, low-fat foods • Open discussion of any topic the group chooses	• Demographics • Diabetes knowledge • Diabetes-related health beliefs • Glycosylated hemoglobin • Fasting blood glucose • Systolic and diastolic blood pressure • Total cholesterol: 　HDL cholesterol 　LDL cholesterol • Triglycerides • Home glucose monitoring

Source: Brown, S. A., Garcia, A. A., Kouzekanani, K., Hanis, C. L. (2002). Culturally competent diabetes self-management education for Mexican Americans. *Diabetes Care 25*, 259–268. Reprinted with permission from the American Diabetes Association.

for further description of the intervention). These materials were culturally competent regarding language, diet, social emphasis, family participation, and inclusion of cultural beliefs. Problem-solving skills were emphasized. The experimental group showed significantly lower levels of HbA1C and fasting blood glucose and higher diabetes knowledge scores at 6 and 12 months (Brown, Garcia, Kouzekanani, Hanis, 2002).

In general, reaching underserved populations for SM preparation requires the kind of extension of usual practice described above. Maintenance of outcomes depends on linking patients to community SM support resources or integration of similar supports into primary care. Because session attendance is variable with this population, proactive calls from a nurse educator have generally proved very effective (Eakin, Bull, Glasgow, Mason, 2002).

DIABETES PROBLEM-SOLVING MEASURE FOR ADOLESCENTS (DPSMA; FIGURE 9.1)

DPSMA is a structured interview-based instrument that examines how adolescents with type 1 diabetes solve diabetes-related SM problems. Adolescence is frequently a time of deteriorating glycemic control. Adherence, which is especially important given the findings of the DCCT, is partly responsible. Tight control involves making adjustments in the regimen, which relies heavily on effective problem-solving strategies. The key management problems perceived by adolescents and their parents include insulin adjustment, diet management, glucose monitoring, recognizing and responding to glycemic deviations, and psychosocial issues.

These problems were encapsulated in 17 critical incidents. They were reviewed for content validity by a panel of experts. The experts also created correct and incorrect responses according to three levels of scoring: (1) recognizing the problem, (2) taking appropriate steps to solve it, and (3) following up on the action to determine effectiveness.

The total score range is 0–34, with a response being considered partially correct for two of the three parts. Interrater reliability was .8–.9, and test-retest reliability was .6–.7. The total

Diabetes Problem-Solving Measure for Adolescents

Vignette	Scoring		
	2 Points	1 Point	0 Points
1. Imagine that you're with your friends at McDonald's and you see something that you're really tempted to eat. The tempting food is not on your diet but you really want to eat it. Your friends are able to order anything they want. You're tired of not getting to eat what you want. What would you do? [If eat food, continue to prompt to cover what might do later in day. If stay with regimen, go to Question 2. Ask next question only if stayed with regimen in Question 1.]	Test and adjust regimen, or resist temptation, follow meal plan, and monitor blood glucose more often	Adjust regimen without testing, or testing without adjustments, or delayed/insufficient adjustment	Inappropriate adjustment or no adjustment
2. Let's say you decided to go ahead and eat the tempting food we just talked about. Then what would you do?	Test more frequently to monitor glucose and make necessary management plans if high	Adjust regimen without testing, or testing without adjustments, or delayed/insufficient adjustment	Inappropriate adjustment or no adjustment
3. It's Saturday, and you've overslept. It's 11:00 A.M. and you normally would have taken your insulin four hours ago. What would you do? Would you make any changes later in the day?	Test and take appropriate insulin (more regular, less NPH) and eat and test more frequently to monitor blood glucose	Modify meal plan without testing, or testing without adjustments, or delayed/insufficient adjustment, or 2-point response without testing	Inappropriate adjustment or no adjustment
4. It's just before dinner and you've checked your blood sugar. It's higher than it should be. What would you do?	Take more insulin, reduce food intake, or exercise and test more often to monitor response	2-point response without immediate or follow-up blood glucose testing	Inappropriate adjustment or no adjustment
5. You're about to go out on Saturday morning with some friends. You really have no idea what time you'll get to eat lunch, and you know that you need to do something to keep your blood sugar from getting out of control. You expect to get home around dinnertime. What would you do?	Test and carry money or food	Have lunch without testing or reduce insulin and skip meal	Skip meal without adjustment or inappropriate adjustment

FIGURE 9.1

181

	Scoring		
Vignette	**2 Points**	**1 Point**	**0 Points**
6. Imagine that you're at the movies and you begin to have problems seeing the screen. Everything looks blurry and you're seeing double. You're feeling shaky and weak. What would you do?	Test **and** manage appropriately	Regimen adjustment without testing, **or** testing without adjustment, **or** delayed/ insufficient adjustment	Inappropriate adjustment **or** no adjustment
7. It is September and the school year just started. You attend gym class every afternoon, and in class you play soccer. Although you really like soccer, you're not used to running around that much. You've noticed that your sugars are always kind of low after gym class, around 60. What would you do?	Test before gym **and** eat snack to cover extra activity, **or** adjust morning regimen to prevent low blood glucose	Modify meal plan without testing, **or** testing without adjustments, **or** delayed/ insufficient adjustment	Inappropriate adjustment **or** no adjustment
8. It's lunchtime at school. You know you are supposed to test your blood sugar, but you don't have much time and it is really a bother to test. What would you do?	Test as required	Delay test	Omit test
9. Lately you're feeling really down and discouraged about having diabetes. You try to distract yourself by thinking about other things. But it just doesn't make you feel any better. You don't know where to turn. What would you do?	Seek social support	Use nonsocial outlet to relieve distress	Do nothing **or** cope maladaptively
10. Lately when you've gone out with your friends you have been eating too much and your sugars have been high. You plan to go out with your friends tonight and you don't want to feel embarrassed and different from them by not eating like them, yet you want to keep your sugars in better control. What would you do?	Test and make regimen adjustment, **or** resist temptation and follow diet regimen	Adjust regimen without testing, **or** testing without adjustment, **or** delayed/ insufficient adjustment	Inappropriate adjustment **or** no adjustment
11. You went to sleep at 11:00 P.M. All of a sudden, you wake up at 2:00 A.M., which you don't usually do. You feel very hungry and you can't really focus your eyes. What would you do?	Test **and** manage appropriately	Treat as low blood glucose without testing	Inappropriate treatment **or** no treatment

FIGURE 9.1   (continued)

Vignette	Scoring		
	2 Points	1 Point	0 Points
12. You are going to spend Thanksgiving Day with your relatives. They always serve lots of good food, but most of the food they serve is not on your meal plan. In the past, you found it hard to keep from overeating. What would you do?	Test and adjust regimen, or resist temptation and follow meal plan	Adjust regimen without testing, or testing without adjustments, or delayed/ insufficient adjustment	Inappropriate adjustment or no adjustment
13. You are going to the clinic at 4:00 P.M., so you know that your dinner will be later than usual. What would you do?	Adhere to regimen scheduling, or monitor blood glucose and treat any deviation accordingly	Modify regimen without testing, or testing without adjustments, or delayed/ insufficient adjustment	Inappropriate adjustment or no adjustment
14. You are at a party with your friends. Everyone is drinking regular pop and mixed alcohol drinks. If you wanted to have a drink, other than a diet drink, what would you do?	Not consume alcohol, or test blood glucose prior to drinking and make appropriate adjustment	Modify regimen without testing, or testing without adjustments, or delayed/ insufficient adjustment	Inappropriate adjustment or no adjustment
15. Imagine that you have just awakened at your normal time in the morning. The first thing you do is check your blood sugar. It is low. What would you do?	Treat low and test to monitor outcome	Modify regimen without testing, or testing without adjustments, or delayed/ insufficient adjustment	Inappropriate adjustment or no adjustment
16. Every morning for the past week your blood sugar has been low when you checked it just before you took your insulin shot. What would you do?	Adjust evening regimen or seek medical advice	Treat low blood glucose but not low blood glucose pattern	Inappropriate adjustment or no adjustment
17. Every morning for the past week your blood sugar has been too high. What would you do?	Adjust evening regimen or seek medical advice	Treat high blood glucose but not high blood glucose pattern	Inappropriate adjustment or no adjustment

Source: Cook, S., Aikens, J. E., Berry, C. A., McNabb, W. L. (2001). Development of the Diabetes Problem-Solving Measure for Adolescents. *The Diabetes Educator 27*, 865–874.

FIGURE 9.1 *(continued)*

score correlated positively with adherence to SE, quality of life, and metabolic control, providing evidence of construct validity. No evidence on sensitivity to treatment effects following an educational intervention on diabetes problem solving could be located (Cook, Aikens, Berry, McNabb, 2001).

INSTRUMENT TO MEASURE DIABETES MANAGEMENT
SELF-EFFICACY IN ADOLESCENTS WITH TYPE I DIABETES
(FIGURE 9.2)

SE is believed to influence SM of diabetes with different types of the disease and different age groups. This instrument was developed both in English and Dutch to measure SE in adolescents with type 1 diabetes mellitus. Items were generated through focus group interviews and their relevance was judged by a team of experts on SM behavior in adolescents. The following situations seemed to be particularly difficult for adolescents: not taking candies, adjusting insulin doses or meals in stressful periods such as exams or sports, and making extra checks of blood glucose when taking a long trip or when sleeping a long time. These difficult situations were integrated into the instrument. Also represented were the different behavioral domains of diabetes SM: injecting insulin (six items); nutrition (nine items); regulating diabetes (seven items); hypo- and hyperglycemia (five items); and three general items about having diabetes.

A five-point Likert response scale was used. The SE scores were summed and divided by the total number of items to indicate the strength of perceived SE for different levels of performance. Higher scores showed less SE. The measure of internal consistency was .86. An exploratory factor analysis produced two factors that reflect general and more difficult SM situations (Moens, Grypdonck, van der Bijl, 2001).

LITERACY ASSESSMENT TOOL FOR PERSONS WITH DIABETES
(LAD) (FIGURE 9.3)

It is difficult to identify patients with low literacy. LAD was developed as a word recognition test composed of three graded word lists specific to diabetes, given in ascending difficulty. This instrument measures patients' ability to pronounce terms they would encounter during clinic visits and in reading menu and self-care instructions. Because LAD can be administered in three to five minutes, patients with diabetes can be quickly screened to determine their ability to read the material that is necessary for them to understand their diet and medical condition. The raw score is scaled to a reading grade level. The

Diabetes Management Self-Efficacy Scale for Adolescents with Type 1 Diabetes

Instructions

As a person with diabetes, you have to perform several activities on a day-to-day basis to manage your diabetes as well as possible. Some of these activities are performed more successfully than others. The purpose of this scale is to let us know how convinced you are in performing all these activities.

The 26 items of the scale have to do with managing your diabetes. All the items have to be answered by you personally, because we are interested in your opinion about your diabetes management! There are no good or bad answers.

It is of great importance that you read the items carefully and complete all the items.

Every item has five response alternatives. Select the alternative (by marking the response alternative you have selected) that best represents your opinion. Attention: No more than one answer per item is allowed.

For example

I'm convinced that I am able to repair a flat tire on my bicycle:

( ) yes, surely

( ) probably yes

( ) maybe yes, maybe no

(X) probably not

( ) no, surely not

If you answer "probably not" (the fourth response alternative), then mark the fourth alternative as shown in the example above.

Scale Items

1. I'm convinced that I am able to continually alternate my insulin injection places.
2. I'm convinced that I can inject my insulin in all situations.
3. I'm convinced that I can react correctly in case of forgetting sometimes to inject insulin.
4. I'm convinced that I can inject my insulin at the right time of the day.
5. I'm convinced that I am able to do an extra check of my blood sugar when out for a long time and not able to take my meal directly.
6. I'm convinced that I am able to adjust my insulin dose and/or diet when going in for sports.
7. I'm convinced that I can choose what to eat or not.
8. I'm convinced that I can adjust my insulin dose in relation to my nutritional needs.

FIGURE 9.2

Scale Items

9. There are two versions of this question:

Question intended for persons who inject insulin one or two times a day:

9a. I'm convinced that I am able to eat all the required meals and snacks.

Question intended for persons who inject insulin three or four times a day:

9b. I'm convinced that I am able to perform extra blood sugar control in case of skipping a meal or eating at a later point in time.

10. I'm convinced that I can refuse sugared candies when offered by friends.

11. I'm convinced that I am able to keep my diet when going to a party.

12. I'm convinced that I am able to take sufficient exercise regularly or do sports.

13. I'm convinced that I am able to adjust my diet and/or insulin dose correctly when getting up late.

14. I'm convinced that I can carry out regular consults with my physician for diabetes control.

15. I'm convinced that I am able to check my blood sugar as many times as advised by my physician or the diabetes team, and not only when I feel that my blood sugar is too high or too low.

16. I'm convinced that I am able to discuss the results of my blood sugar tests with my physician or with somebody on the diabetes team, even when they are not satisfactory.

17. I'm convinced that I can feel when my blood sugar is too low.

18. I'm convinced that I am able to take Dextro's (or sugar, cookie, Coke, . . .) with me when I go out.

19. I'm convinced that I can feel when my blood sugar is too high.

20. I'm convinced that I am able to eat a snack in the classroom in case of a hypo, even when my classmates are watching.

21. I'm convinced that I am able to adjust my insulin dose and/or diet when having exams or difficult tests.

22. I'm convinced that I am able to eat exactly sufficient food in case of a hypo.

23. I'm convinced that I dare to tell at a new school that I have diabetes.

24. I'm convinced that I am able to tell my friends what I have to do and not do because of my diabetes.

25. I'm convinced that I can adjust my insulin dose correctly in case of illness.

26. I'm convinced that I am able to manage my diabetes when staying with friends as well as when I am at home.

Source: Moens, A., Grypdonck, M. H. F., van der Bijl, J. J. (2001). The development and psychometric testing of an instrument to measure diabetes management self-efficacy in adolescents with type 1 diabetes. *Scholarly Inquiry for Nursing Practice 15*, 223–233. Used by permission of Springer Publishing Company, Inc., New York.

FIGURE 9.2 *(continued)*

majority of the terms are on a fourth-grade reading level, with the remaining words ranging from the sixth- through sixteenth-grade levels. LAD is significantly correlated with other literacy tests, supporting its validity. Test-retest reliability is .92 (Nath, Sylvester, Yasek, Gunel, 2001).

Literacy Assessment for Diabetes (LAD)

Patient Name/Number _____ Birth date _____

Date _____ Clinic _____ Examiner _____

List 1		List 2		List 3	
eat	____	**thirst**	____	**artery**	____
eet		thŭrst		'art-tĕ-ree or 'ar-tree	
pill	____	**exercise**	____	**biosynthetic**	____
pĭl		'ek-sir-sīz		bī-ō-sin-'thet-ik	
eye	____	**exchange**	____	**abnormal**	____
ī		iks-'chänj		ab-'nor-muhl	
fat	____	**direction**	____	**cholesterol**	____
fat		duh-'rek-shŭn		kah-'les-tuh-rawl or rōl	
milk	____	**hospital**	____	**glycogen**	____
milk		'hos-pit-uhl		'gli-kuh-jĕn	
sugar	____	**calorie**	____	**nephropathy**	____
'shoo-gĕr		'kal-uh-ree		ni-'frap-uh-thē	
lunch	____	**colon**	____	**prescription**	____
lunch		'kō-luhn		pri-'skrip-shuhn	
meals	____	**urination**	____	**pregnancy**	____
meelz		yoor-uh-'nay-shun		'preg-nuhn-see	
kidney	____	**vision**	____	**ketones**	____
'kid-nee		'vizh-un		'kee-tōnz	
drink	____	**protein**	____	**ketoacidosis**	____
drink		'prō-teen		kee-tō-ass-ih-'dō-sus	
nurse	____	**vegetable**	____	**pancreas**	____
nurs		'vej-tuh-bul		'pan-kree-uhs	
fiber	____	**snack**	____	**hypoglycemia**	____
'fi-bĕr		snak		hī-pō-gl ī-'see-mee-uh	
fruits	____	**cereal**	____	**atherosclerosis**	____
frootz		'ser-ee-ul		ath-uh-rō-skluh-'rō-sis	
supper	____	**injection**	____	**occupation**	____
'sŭp-ĕr		in-'jek-shun		ok-yoo-'pay-shuhn	

FIGURE 9.3

187

List 1		List 2		List 3	
bread	_____	glucose	_____	triglycerides	_____
bred		'gloo-kōs		trī-'glis-uh-rīds	
heart	_____	breakfast	_____	emergency	_____
hart		'brek-fuhst		ih-'mūr-juhn-see	
blood	_____	insulin	_____	communication	_____
bluhd		'in-suh-lin		kuh-mū-nuh-'kā-shuhn	
stress	_____	alcohol	_____	hemoglobin	_____
stress		'al-kuh-hall		'hē-muh-glō-buhn	
meat	_____	medication	_____	endocrinologist	_____
meet		med-ah-'kā-shuhn		en-duh-krih-'nawl-uh-jist	
doctor	_____	symptom	_____	retinopathy	_____
'dok-tūr		'simp-tuhm		ret-ehn-'op-uh-thē	

Raw Score	Estimation of Grade Level	Score
0–20	Fourth grade and below (Oral instructions should be given repeatedly with visual assistance.)	List 1 _____ List 2 _____ List 3 _____
21–40	Fifth–ninth grade level	
41–60	Ninth grade and above	Raw Score _____

Instructions for Administering the Literacy Assessment for Diabetes

The Literacy Assessment for Diabetes (LAD) is a screening instrument to assess an adult patient's ability to read ordinary nutritional and medical terms as well as those terms specific to diabetes. The purpose of this test is to indicate relevant literacy information to those medical personnel who assist diabetic patients in understanding nutritional and medical instructions.

Word Reading

Subjects are to pronounce 60 words, arranged in three columns in order of increasing complexity. Half of the words are at the fourth-grade level, the rest range from sixth- through sixteenth-grade level. The word list used by the administrator of the test provides space for scoring responses and a pronunciation guide.

The LAD consists of a laminated reading list from which subjects read, and the same list with a pronunciation key for the administrator of the test. The administrator should have a clipboard and pencil when testing subjects.

The test is to be administered one-on-one, rather than in a group setting. The LAD tests the subject's ability to recognize words — not the subject's speech or diction. The LAD counts certain nonstandard pronunciations as correct if the subject uses the nonstandard pronunciation consistently throughout the test. Examples of nonstandard pronunciation include English as a second language, speech impediments, or use of a nonstandard English dialect. The LAD is designed for use with adults.

FIGURE 9.3 (continued)

The examiner's copy of the LAD provides the correct pronunciations just below the words. The examiner should familiarize himself or herself with this pronunciation guide before administering the test and should follow the pronunciation guide as he or she scores the test. The examiner's copy should not be visible to the subject. Should the subject be curious about the correct pronunciation of words, this should be deferred until after the test is completed.

Many low- or non-literate subjects are very sensitive about their inability to read and should be treated at all times with courtesy and respect. Their inability to read should not be treated as blameworthy. Before beginning testing, make sure that those subjects who need eyeglasses or contact lenses are wearing them for the test.

Directions for Word Reading

1. Give the patient a laminated copy of the LAD and score answers on the unlaminated (or administrator's) copy. Hold your copy so that it does not distract your testee.

SAY: *Would you please read **aloud** as many words as you can from the lists. Start with the first word on List 1, and read down the list. When you have finished with the first list, start at the top of the next list, and so on. When you come to a word you cannot read, try your best or say "pass" and go on to the next word.*

2. If the patient takes more than five seconds on a word, say "*pass*" and point to the next word, if necessary, to move the patient along. If the patient passes five or more times allow him or her to attempt only words they know.

Directions for Scoring

3. Place a plus (+) after each correctly pronounced word, a zero (0) after each mispronounced word, and a minus (−) after words not attempted. A word that the patient self-corrects is counted as a correct word and marked with a plus (+).

4. Count the number of correct words (+) for each of the three lists and record the number in the "SCORE" box. Total the numbers and write the total in the corresponding blanks. The raw score is the total of the three lists. The raw score can then be converted to a reading grade level using the conversion table printed on the tool score sheet.

This educational tool was developed and funded through a grant from the West Virginia Diabetes Council Program, West Virginia Bureau of Public Health, West Virginia Department of Health and Human Resources, and West Virginia University. © 2000 WVU

Source: Nath, C. R., Sylvester, S. T., Yasek, V., Gunel, E. (2001). Development and validation of a literacy assessment tool for persons with diabetes. *The Diabetes Educator 27*, 857–864.

FIGURE 9.3   *(continued)*

References

Bonnet, C., Gagnayre, R., d'Ivernois, J. F. (2001). Difficulties of diabetic patients in learning about their illness. *Patient Education & Counseling 42*, 159–164.

Brown, S. A., Garcia, A. A., Kouzekanani, K., Hanis, C. L. (2002). Culturally competent diabetes self-management education for Mexican Americans. *Diabetes Care 25*, 259–268.

Calle-Pascual, A. L., et al. (2002). A preventative foot care programme for people with diabetes with different stages of neuropathy. *Diabetes Research and Clinical Practice 57,* 111–117.

Cook, S., Aikens, J. E., Berry, C. A., McNabb, W. L. (2001). Development of the Diabetes Problem-Solving Measure for Adolescents. *The Diabetes Educator 27,* 865–874.

Cox, D. J., Gonder-Frederick, L. A., Kovatchev, B. P., Clarke, W. L. (2001). Self-treatment of hypoglycemia while driving. *Diabetes Research and Clinical Practice 54,* 17–26.

Delamater, A. M., et al. (2001). Psychosocial therapies in diabetes. *Diabetes Care 24,* 1286–1292.

Eakin, E. G., Bull, S. S., Glasgow, R. E., Mason, M. (2002). Reaching those most in need: A review of diabetes self-management interventions in disadvantaged populations. *Diabetes Metabolism Research and Reviews 18,* 26–35.

Fiel, E. G., Glasgow, R. E., Boles, S., McKay, H. G. (2000). Who participates in Internet-based self-management programs? A study among novice computer users in a primary care setting. *The Diabetes Educator 26,* 806–811.

Glasgow, R. E., et al. (2002). Self-management aspects of the improving chronic care breakthrough series: Implementation with diabetes and heart failure teams. *Annals of Behavioral Medicine 24*(2), 80–87.

Gonder-Frederick, L. A., Cox, D. J., Ritterband, L. R. (2002). Diabetes and behavioral medicine: The second decade. *Journal of Consulting and Clinical Psychology 70,* 611–625.

Hampson, S. E., Glasgow, R. E., Strycker, L. A. (2000). Belief versus feelings: A comparison of personal models and depression for predicting multiple outcomes in diabetes. *British Journal of Health Psychology 5,* 27–40.

Heisler, M. B., Reynard R., Hayward, R. A., Smith, S. M., Kerr, E. A. (2002). The relative importance of physician communication, participatory decision making, and patient understanding in diabetes self-management. *Journal of General Internal Medicine 17,* 243–252.

Howorka, K., et al. (2000). Empowering diabetes out-patients with structured education: Short-term and long-term effects of functional insulin treatment on perceived control over diabetes. *Journal of Psychosomatic Research 48,* 37–44.

McKay, H. G., King, D., Eakin, E. G., Seeley, J. R., Glasgow, R. E. (2001). The Diabetes Network Internet-based physical activity intervention. *Diabetes Care 24,* 1328–1334.

McMurray, S. D., Johnson, G., Davis, S., McDougall, K. (2002). Diabetes education and care management significantly improve patient outcomes in the dialysis unit. *American Journal of Kidney Diseases 40,* 566–575.

Mensing, C., et al. (2000). National standards for diabetes self-management education. *Diabetes Care 23,* 682–689.

Moens, A., Grypdonck, M. H. F., van der Bijl, J. J. (2001). The development and psychometric testing of an instrument to measure diabetes management self-efficacy in adolescents with type 1 diabetes. *Scholarly Inquiry for Nursing Practice 15,* 223–233.

Nath, C. R., Sylvester, S. T., Yasek, V., Gunel, E. (2001). Development and validation of a literacy assessment tool for persons with diabetes. *The Diabetes Educator 27,* 857–864.

Norris, S. L., et al. (2002). Increasing diabetes self-management education in community settings: A systematic review. *American Journal of Preventive Medicine 22*(4S), 39–66.

Norris, S. L., Engelgau, M. M., Narayan, K. M. V. (2001). Effectiveness of self-management training in type 2 diabetes. *Diabetes Care 24,* 561–422.

Norris, S. L., Lau, J., Smith, S. J., Schmid, C. H., Engelgau, M. M. (2002). Self-management education for adults with type 2 diabetes. *Diabetes Care 25,* 1159–1171.

Parchman, M. L., Pugh, J. A., Noel, P. H., Larme, A. C. (2002). Continuity of care, self-management behaviors and glucose control in patients with type 2 diabetes. *Medical Care 40,* 137–144.

Paterson, B., Thorne, S. (2000a). Developmental evolution of expertise in diabetes self-management. *Clinical Nursing Research 9,* 402–419.

Paterson, B., Thorne, S. (2000b). Expert decision making in relation to unanticipated blood glucose levels. *Research in Nursing & Health 23,* 147–157.

Peeples, M., Mulcahy, K., Tomky, D., Weaver, T. (2001). The conceptual framework of the National Diabetes Education Outcomes System (NDEOS). *The Diabetes Educator 27,* 547–562.

Piette, J. D., et al. (2000). Do automated calls with nurse follow-up improve self-care and glycemic control among vulnerable patients with diabetes? *American Journal of Medicine 108,* 20–27.

Piette, J. D., Glasgow, R. E. (2001). Education and home glucose monitoring. In Gerstein, H. C., Haynes, R. B., eds. *Evidence-based diabetes care.* Hamilton: B. C. Decker.

Renders, C. M., et al. (2001). Interventions to improve the management of diabetes in primary care, outpatient, and community settings. *Diabetes Care 24,* 1821–1833.

Roman, S. H., Chassin, M. R. (2001). Windows of opportunity to improve diabetes care when patients with diabetes are hospitalized for other conditions. *Diabetes Care 24,* 1371–1376.

Schilling, L. S., Grey, M., Knafl, K. A. (2002). The concept of self-management of type 1 diabetes in children and adolescents: An evolutionary concept analysis. *Journal of Advanced Nursing 37,* 87–99.

Schillinger, D., et al. (2002). Association of health literacy with diabetes outcomes. *Journal of the American Medical Association 288,* 475–482.

Sinclair, A. J., Girling, A. J., Bayer, A. J. (2000). Cognitive dysfunction in older subjects with diabetes mellitus: Impact on diabetes self-management and use of care services. *Diabetes Research and Clinical Practice 50,* 203–212.

U.S. Department of Health and Human Services. (2000). *Healthy People 2010.* Washington, D.C.

Williams, M. V., Baker, D. W., Parker, R. M., Nurss, J. R. (1998). Relationship of functional health literacy to patients' knowledge of their chronic disease. *Archives of Internal Medicine 158,* 166–172.

Yawn, B., Zyzanski, S. J., Goodwin, M. A., Gotler, R. S., Stange, K. C. (2001). Is diabetes treated as an acute or chronic illness in community family practice? *Diabetes Care 24,* 1390–1396.

10

Summary and Next Steps

 Evidence of the importance of SM preparation has been presented throughout this book. Likewise, this book has offered evidence of the primitive level of development of this field and the low priority on its support. This situation persists even though for some diseases SM benefit is comparable to that of pharmacologic interventions, for which there is ample support.

This situation is based on certain questionable assumptions:

1. Available SM preparation should be limited to diseases and symptoms for which there is a recognized moderately efficacious medical treatment (e.g., diabetes, asthma). Individuals with diseases or symptoms lacking a less efficacious medical treatment must also self-manage, frequently without even a basic knowledge of their situations, and derive their own SM with very little help (e.g., epilepsy, multiple sclerosis, Parkinson's disease, urinary incontinence, sickle cell disease). If the health care system were guided more by patient/family needs and driven less by physicians' desires to assure compliance to medical treatment, SM preparation would be available for all chronic diseases and symptoms. Interestingly, many patients for whom SM is not "prescribed" are doing portions of it anyway, frequently without direction and potentially incorrectly.

2. If SM is not working, the problem must be patient noncompliance, not the quality of the medical regimen, even though deviance from well-established standards of medical practice is legion. Routine quality control should pick up and correct errors in SM preparation as well as true patient SM errors.

3. SM is an add-on to routine medical management including use of pharmaceuticals. Only recently have comparisons assessed the value added to disease outcomes by SM preparation versus those obtained through other modalities such as pharmaceuticals. Ongoing expenses related to pharmaceutical care are accepted; the continuing education necessary for adequate SM is not. In part, this discrepancy reflects a widespread misconception of what is necessary to develop and maintain SM skills (continued SE and problem solving as opposed to a single shot of knowledge).

The previous chapters suggest certain conclusions about the state of the field. First, SM preparation has been significantly underdeveloped and lacks appropriate investment. While the reason for this lag is not immediately clear, several interpretations could be made. Perhaps the most likely is the ideological bent of the medical model of health care, which focuses on diagnosis and biological treatment of disease, yet ignores psychosocial interventions. The poor, the elderly, and the uneducated suffer disproportionately from this state of affairs. These groups are more likely to have chronic diseases and require more sustained interventions to achieve and maintain competent SM.

A second, well-recognized conclusion is that the structure of the current health care system does not well serve patients with chronic illness, including those trying to self-manage. Continuity of care is disrupted by boundaries between elements of the health care system. In addition, settings where patients with chronic disease for whom SM preparation has never been available or in whom SM has failed — such as EDs — don't offer the preparation that these patients need to become competent self-managers. Disease management programs have shown some success in bridging these boundaries and offering these services but are available for only a small portion of patients and are driven primarily by the goal of containing costs.

The current ideological bent and health care system allow health professionals to avoid the hard work of being accountable for successful SM preparation and other elements of chronic disease control. Most of the well-developed areas of SM preparation (e.g., diabetes, asthma, arthritis) have research bases that show the efficacy and effectiveness of SM in selected populations. This research demonstrates that patients can be prepared to control their disease so they can regain productive lives. Unfortunately, this service remains largely unavailable to them and even less available to poor, minority populations with limited literacy. Sharon Brown's work cited in Chapter 9 shows that successful culturally appropriate SM preparation can be provided to these individuals, although it appears that a sustained, potent intervention is necessary. It should be noted that it will be impossible to meet the *Healthy People 2010* population-level goals without assisting the poor and the old.

While measurement instruments exist for some important intermediate outcomes such as knowledge level and SE, means by which to assess the complex reasoning and behavioral responses needed to self-manage a chronic disease are not available. For this reason, informal clinical but not quantitative approaches to evaluate a patient's capabilities are the norm, limiting the setting of standards and benchmarks for adequate SM preparation.

By all standards of professional practice, lack of competent SM preparation is substandard care and unethical. Yet, this situation has generated neither a sense of moral outrage nor potent political movements to force reform, perhaps in part because those most dramatically affected tend to be poor and disenfranchised. Largely, the status quo is accepted as the way things have to be. Evidence for this view is that virtually no adequate practice standards exist for SM preparation.

A set of conclusions may also be drawn about SM preparation itself. First, the lack of a common language and a taxonomy by which to describe SM preparation interventions presents a problem. Second, a paucity of instruments is available to measure SM skills and judgments, not just SE or beliefs. These two deficits seriously hamper efforts to benchmark or improve quality or even to communicate to health professionals how to do SM preparation.

Most of the diseases reviewed in this book use problem solving and SE as the theoretical base for their interventions. Pain is the only area where assessment and alteration of false beliefs is used. In a number of areas, phases of readiness for SM preparation/adaptation to the disease are described; it is not clear how frequently such frameworks are used to guide interventions. Developmental phases have been described in the chapters on diabetes, arthritis, pain, and asthma. In some disease entities, such as HIV/AIDS and hypertension, SM preparation is atheoretical.

In only a few fields, such as arthritis, are well-developed and validated models of SM preparation available. In some diseases, SM means primarily self-monitoring; in others, it also includes self-treatment. Reasons for this discrepancy seem to have more to do with custom than with a clear set of criteria for the amount of responsibility that patients might take.

The degree to which symptoms and responses are idiosyncratic to individuals is generally underappreciated. In part, this is undoubtedly due to incomplete knowledge about the causes of disease (that is, why it is chronic). It is insufficient to give a patient a list of standard symptoms and expect that they fit that individual's particular experience. In addition, conflict in regimens from multiple comorbidities is frequently not addressed.

The economic impact of SM preparation has not been thoroughly addressed, yet the stakes are huge: More than 75% of all U.S. health care expenditures are related to treatment of chronic disease. By 2020, nearly half of the population is projected to have at least one chronic condition (Wolff, Starfield, Anderson, 2002).

Successful chronic illness care depends heavily on nonphysician personnel to conduct routine assessments, provide support and preparation for SM, and assure follow-up. At the same time, institutional roles for these providers heavily constrain them in carrying out these roles. An example of an arrangement that dealt successfully with this problem may be found in asthma (Chapter 8). Patients whose pharmacists noted that they were using excessive amounts of bronchodilator therapy were referred directly to asthma SM preparation centers, as opposed to being required to go through physician gatekeepers or ignoring warning signs of the problem. To date, there has been very little study of incorporation of SM preparation into regular professional visits; most of the research studies separate SM preparation programs. Nevertheless, health care systems in Europe have successfully trained and certified health professionals (a necessary step) and developed practices to integrate SM preparation into ongoing primary and specialty care.

SM preparation is one of several kinds of patient education, which differ in the outcome desired and, therefore, the methods to be used. The outcomes desired from SM are competent management by the patient/family of the disease or symptom and as good a quality of life as possible. The complexity of the learning requires methods such as active practice with problem solving based on full knowledge of the management regimen, strong SE and decision making, and social negotiation skills. Other purposes for which patient education is used include preparation for procedures, rehabilitative education, caregiving, self-diagnosis to obtain care such as for myocardial infarction or stroke, adjustment to the diagnosis or illness, and different kinds of preparation. There is no such thing as general-purpose patient education.

New Approaches to Self-Management

Some new research findings point the way toward how SM might eventually be practiced. Some enhance the theoretical base, whereas others develop SM approaches for diseases that do not currently have them.

For example, the transtheoretical model describes a way to match interventions to the patient's readiness to change. Assessment methods by which to accomplish this sorting appear in Figures 10.1 and 10.2 and can be adapted to other diseases (Doherty, James and Roberts, 2000).

197

Please look at the statements below. Which one best describes how you feel right now about improving your diabetes self management?

Which statement
fits for you?
Check [√] one only.

There is no need for me to think about my diabetes.	☐
I don't want to think about my diabetes.	☐
It's a waste of time thinking about my diabetes.	☐
I am weighing up the advantages and disadvantages of improving my diabetes.	☐
Sometimes I think I might benefit from improving my diabetes but haven't decided yet.	☐
I have definitely decided to improve my diabetes.	☐
I am planning how to improve my diabetes.	☐
I am actually trying to improve my diabetes and started to do something about it.	☐
I have managed to improve my diabetes; I just need to keep it going.	☐
I have now improved my diabetes and I am trying to avoid slipping back into my old ways.	☐
I have given up trying to improve my diabetes.	☐
I have not been able to keep the change going.	☐

Scoring key: The first three items would suggest the individual was precontemplative. Items 4 and 5 refer to contemplation, 6 and 7 determination, and 8 suggests early action. Nine and 10 would indicate attempts at maintenance, with 11 and 12 indicating relapse.

FIGURE 10.1   A method to aid assessment of stage of change for diabetes self-management

Ulcerative colitis is managed mainly by regular outpatient reviews. In a randomized controlled trial, Robinson, Thompson, Wilkin, and Roberts (2001) tested an intervention in which patients monitored and treated their symptoms, obtained advice when necessary, and referred themselves to the hospital when they needed treatment outside agreed-upon guidelines. While ulcerative colitis is not usually self-managed, in this study patients so managed had their relapses treated much more quickly, had decreased physician visits, and did not suffer increased morbidity in comparison with a usual-treatment group. Intervention

Being more active?

Please look at the six pictures and statements below. Which best describes how you feel right now about being more active?

Which picture fits for you? Check (√) one only.

☐ *Staying put*

☐ *Wondering where to go*

☐ *Planning*

☐ *Taking the first steps*

☐ *I've made it thus far*

☐ *I'm back to where I started*

Which statement fits for you? Check (√) one only.

There is no need for me to think about being more active. ☐

I don't want to think about being more active. ☐

It's a waste of time thinking about being more active. ☐

I am weighing up the advantages and disadvantages of becoming more active. ☐

Sometimes I think I might benefit from becoming more active, but haven't decided yet. ☐

I have definitely decided to be more active. ☐

I am planning how to be more active. ☐

I am actually trying to be more active. ☐

I know that I should do more activity and have started to do something about it. ☐

I have managed to be more active; I just need to keep it going. ☐

I am now more active and trying to avoid slipping back into my old ways. ☐

I have given up trying to be more active. ☐

I have not been able to keep the change going. ☐

Source: Doherty, Y., James, P., Roberts, S. (2000). Stage of change counseling. In Snoek, F. J., Skinner, T. C., eds. *Psychology in diabetes care.* New York: John Wiley and Sons.

FIGURE 10.2 An assessment method using stage-specific pictures and statements for a specific behavior

patients were asked to make a clinic appointment only if self-treatment did not improve their symptoms within seven days, if relapses returned when treatment decreased, if more than two courses of oral prednisolone were needed within a year, if rectal bleeding occurred between relapses, if patients experienced an unexplained weight loss, or if they wanted a consultation. The appropriateness of self-treatment was assessed from patient diaries.

Another example of an approach to SM was studied by Brody and colleagues (1999) for age-related macular degeneration (AMD). AMD is the leading cause of incurable blindness and low vision in older adults; one out of five persons aged 65 and older can expect to have some vision loss due to AMD. There is no treatment to restore vision to premorbid levels of acuity and no well-established preventive measures exist. Macular degeneration patients have reported greater life stress, lower satisfaction, and lower activity levels than controls. If they have low vision in both eyes, these patients report significant emotional distress and health-related quality of life. Distress symptoms among patients who still retain functional vision may be better predictors of disability and loss of function than is visual acuity alone.

A six-session SM preparation intervention for AMD incorporated didactic presentation and group problem solving with guided practice. The program included information about the biological processes of AMD, suggestions of ways to maintain or increase activity levels, hands-on demonstrations, and discussions of available visual aids and services. Reevaluation of perceived barriers to independence was encouraged and positive challenges were provided from peers and group leaders. Participants also gained skills training in communicating with others about visual disability and in managing common living problems. Intervention participants experienced substantially decreased psychological distress, increased SE, improved mood, and increased use of vision aids. It is important to note how successful this intervention was in a disease for which no effective medical intervention exists.

No doubt, other comparable examples can be found. Will the health care community "step up to the plate"?

References

Brody, B. L., et al. (1999). Age-related macular degeneration: A randomized clinical trial of a self-management intervention. *Annals of Behavioral Medicine 21,* 322–329.

Doherty, Y., James, P., Roberts, S. (2000). Stage of change counseling. In Snoek, F. J., Skinner, T. C., eds. *Psychology in diabetes care.* New York: John Wiley and Sons.

Robinson, A., Thompson, D. G., Wilkin, D., Roberts, C. (2001). Guided self-management and patient-directed follow-up of ulcerative colitis: A randomised trial. *The Lancet 358,* 976–981.

Wolff, J. L., Starfield, B., Anderson, G. (2002). Prevalence, expenditures and complications of multiple chronic conditions in the elderly. *Archives of Internal Medicine 162,* 2269–2276.

Abbreviations

AED   antiepilepsy drug
AMD   age-related macular degeneration
BAI   breath-activated inhaler
CAPD   continuous ambulatory peritoneal dialysis
COPD   chronic obstructive pulmonary disease
ED   emergency department
EEG   electro-encephalogram
FIT   functional insulin test
HMO   health maintenance organization
INR   international normalized ratio
MA   meta-analysis
MDI   metered-dose inhaler
MRI   magnetic resonance imaging
MS   multiple sclerosis
NSAID   nonsteroidal anti-inflammatory drug
OCD   obsessive-compulsive disorder
PT   prothrombin time
RA   rheumatoid arthritis
RCT   randomized controlled trial
RRT   renal replacement therapy
SE   self-efficacy
SM   self-management
SMBG   self-monitored blood glucose
SMBP   self-management of blood pressure

Index